MW00716725

A CHANCE
MEETING WITH LIFE
Inside an Intensive Care Unit, and Out

A CHANCE MEETING WITH LIFE

Inside an Intensive Care Unit,
and Out

JAN PRICE

Copyright © 2018
Jan Price
A Chance Meeting With Life: Inside an Intensive Care Unit, and Out

All rights reserved. No portion of this book may be reproduced in any form without permission from the publisher, except as permitted by U.S. copyright law.

Available from Amazon and other retail outlets.

Stacks of Books, Inc.
P.O. Box 308
Clifton, Virginia 20124
stacksofbookslife@outlook.com

Book Design by Jeremy V. Fleming
Content Editing by Lisa Canfield
Copy Editing by Stephanie Bond

To view more artwork by:
Christine Cantow Smith
  - www.facebook.com/AuntBeanArtworks

ISBN 978-1-7320994-0-1

Library of Congress Control Number: 2018904314

In dedication to all those in medicine who save lives in such an extraordinary way

CONTENTS

INCOMMUNICADO

The story I am about to tell could be the story of a young girl of twenty-five who has cystic fibrosis. It could be the story of a mother who nearly lost her daughter and didn't, and it could be about what happened to a family. It's really a story about how strong human beings are, and capable, and resilient. Not weak, strong. We can do, and then move forward, and do again. We have to think of ourselves as tough like that young girl of twenty-five was tough, and her mother, too. This is a story about things that should not happen to a person but sometimes they do, and this time did.

Let's get this part out of the way in one sentence, though reading it twice may be necessary.

What is cystic fibrosis?
Cystic fibrosis is a recessive genetic disease

causing the mechanism that releases sodium chloride from the cells to be faulty, imbalancing the body mucuses, making them thick and sticky and harbor bacteria, impacting the sinuses, lungs, and gut, and shortening the life expectancy.

Jackie had always been "followed" at Inova Fairfax Hospital. The medical community does follow people with diseases and that's what it feels like, being followed, necessary, appreciated, dreaded in a way like the diagnosis that would follow Jackie her whole life, though she would not let it get in her way. And then it did. "Inova" is one of those names assigned to a regional medical system and ours is grand, so I always believed, as a mother with hope, it meant "Innovation."

Jackie had several sinus surgeries, the first before age two, a solution for quality-of-life decline, and this time as well. She entered Inova Fairfax Hospital's Heart and Vascular Institute for the sinus surgery expecting to return to work the following week, summer plans set before her. She was living her life as young people do, out on her own and working, yet fragile, lacking endurance, exploring a lung transplant a ways away. Watching her leave on that stretcher entering the sinus surgery, I tucked my head as I'd done before and prayed her lungs would be safe.

I expected a recovery dip in lung function, felt a deep-down dread. Dread is something mothers of children with diseases live with, along with a broken heart held together by determination. The sinus surgery went well, her sinuses were clear and she would feel better, my ever-familiar post-surgery mind mantra. That night, I lay beside Jackie determined that she would get comfortable and move on to healing. Instead, we were transported as a precautionary to an intensive care unit. Her heart rate was up a little and vital signs were off a bit. They did calm down.

Jackie's recovery from sinus surgery remained in order that first while. She was presenting well, animated, leaving the two-day ICU precautionary the following morning. By dinner, a friend was visiting and Jackie called to ask that we come anyhow. Her dad and I did as we had done many times before, yet this time was different. She wasn't used to ICUs, was asking herself why she was there, if she was okay. Once we returned home that night and her dad settled in, I returned to the hospital, hurried along that well-worn path back to Jackie, then with a high fever that quickly flipped before my eyes into an emergency that would take us down a path we'd never traveled.

Dr. Svetolik Djurkovic, pulmonary intensivist, clinical interest: severe infections and respiratory failure, in an all-night effort, pulled Jackie out of respiratory arrest until cardiac arrest was imminent. The heart can only compensate but so much. She tried hard throughout the night to respond to the external ventilator, gasping, "How am I doing, Dad?" He had come during the night as well as her Aunt Anne. We were there, watching, encouraging, hoping, disbelieving. By morning, Jackie plunged by way of doctor into a medically induced coma, and intubation. Before the inevitable, a panicked, "Promise me I'll wake up!" Dr. Djurkovic did, an unconvincing promise Jackie would wake up.

He and his team left Jackie in the care of the ICU team, no longer a precautionary. Our Jackie had that tube inserted into her mouth, down in her airway in one direction, and in the other direction, out of her mouth into a ventilator like a nightstand I'd never seen before with numbers and knobs and beepers and alarms, respiratory therapists and nurses controlling the flow, and multiple pumps by her side on multiple poles, multiple tubes running intravenous infusions into our girl, throwing every intervention at the dangerously high fever and infection that overtook her lungs in the night. They looked at her father and me, we looked at them, the unstated truth Jackie would likely not survive. Jackie did not have a heart attack that night yet did remain in that Coronary Care Unit.

Voice shredded, I called her brother, Byron, in a rush of emotion, "It's Jackie! You have to come now!" He cabbed to the Boston airport, bought a ticket, boarded a plane, and by noon entered Inova Fairfax Hospital's Heart and Vascular Institute just outside of Washington, D.C. That night, Byron created a "Jackie Get Well Update" social media group. "Hey Everyone. My sister isn't doing too well right now and I thought I would throw up this group. We will give updates and please feel free to write good wishes." He continued to describe the sinus surgery and the respiratory free-fall that followed, the intensive care unit, blood pressure and oxygenation issues, and optimism of the doctors and nurses.

No visitors were allowed in that room. Concerted effort to keep Jackie's vital numbers by way of machines in a range of survival remained in that room. It's all about numbers and in this league of medical care, the numbers are in the hands and heads of the doctors, and the hearts. These people don't do this work because they are bored. It's an amazing package, just like the recovery they orchestrated for Jackie and for that, I love them. What is it to love strangers, to love those just met, their voices for the first time heard? The complexity of it all was kept simple for our sake as we placed our daughter further and further into their hands by way of trust.

Jackie was in one-on-one, two-on-one, sometimes three-on-one care, in critical condition due to pneumonia, more specifically a quiet and wicked collusion between bacteria and a rare fungus attempting to overtake her. Her brother wrote again. "Her doctors are hoping her body and a ridiculous amount of antibiotics will fight the infection in this resting state."

An amazing team of intensive care doctors put their minds together as her condition worsened. Our son wrote, "The doctors need complete silence to do their work. Unfortunately, the process will be longer than originally expected. This is brutal." The infection was mean. The medical team's fight was tougher and more determined than the infection was mean. As one nurse said after two hours in the care of Jackie, "Whoa, that was hard." I've always said hard doesn't mean we don't do it. Hard it was, and they did it.

There were a couple of days of constant care and hopeful healing with gentle background music, lights turned down low, us keeping back and quiet. They were doing their best yet her condition worsened. By morning, three days after the first pulmonary free-fall and after a no-worse night, yet another. In a major medical bind, uneventful is good. What was to come was not.

Her dad and I heading down the ICU corridor came upon an emergency and the emergency was ours, a team of prepared, brilliant minds orchestrating a complex plan to save our daughter again, people hurrying about in a blur, determining what to do next, and fast. Jackie's lungs lay inside her on that bed ignited by infection, this second dive to destruction.

Unimaginably, we came upon Dr. James Clayton, pediatric pulmonologist who brought Jackie through childhood starting in the Neonatal Intensive Care Unit. He, too, was coming to visit Jackie, being the amazing soul that he is. I paced half-breathing, half-hearing the voice I trusted all those years. "You watch," he told my husband. "He'll save her. He'll do it. Just watch." Dr. Clayton talked my husband through the crisis madness managed back to sanity by Dr. Christopher King, pulmonologist, intensivist, the mind that saved Jackie that day and in the days to come. I came to call the doctors The Knowing Ones and Dr. King, The Knowingest One, because he saved her at the worst and kept saving her.

It must have taken ten medical professionals to transport her hospital bed to surgery where they put Jackie on an external lung machine, lungs made of metal and hoses, pumps and filters. This extraordinary technology, ECMO, seemed to be new in this particular and terrible circumstance, we thought they said. Who knew? We were no longer on the planet earth. We were in some other universe, one we could not imagine a week before sitting at dinner with Jackie talking about her PowerPoint presentations for work.

The expert in the use of this Extra Corporeal Membrane Oxygenation, so we learned, worked remotely with this Heart and Vascular Institute, traveled there monthly and was there that day. They made a plan. They implemented the plan and for the time, it was working. ECMO gave Jackie a fifty percent chance of surviving as they controlled her vital signs remotely and prepared her for a bilateral lung transplant, a serious surgery with a rough recovery.

None of the expected times had come true as we waited

and as Jackie's condition grew increasingly more complex, yet the goal remained to receive new lungs, wake up one day, spend time again with friends and family. Jackie's Uncle Mark who flew for the military was there that first week, watching those panels on all those machines, like watching those panels in the cockpit of a fighter jet. Jackie was finally stable in a critical-condition kind of way, by way of machine, but stable yet.

We sat there, cousins, aunts and uncles, loved ones, and waited for the doctors to work their long-acquired magic, that ability to save people teetering between life and death. What became pretty were Jackie's vital numbers; what was not pretty was Jackie in that bed moved to the Cardio-Vascular Intensive Care Unit surrounded by yet more tubes running in and out, more panels of numbers flipping up and down, all those machines and that constant medical care. Jackie was not getting up the next day, not going eagerly to Lidl, leaving work to get together with friends and just be Jackie. Jackie was alive and sick as a person could be. We believed she would live. This is the story of how she did.

CHAPTER ONE

IT ALL BEGAN
IN JUNE

The events leading up to Jackie's listing for a lung transplant are both extraordinary and essential. "Incomunicado" will forever be an essential word for me because not only did our daughter overcome incommunicado, but I did as well in being able to tell her story. It all began in June, but it all began first with the Essential Prologue.

Jackie was officially listed for a transplant, seeking a new set of lungs, on life supports, overcoming pneumonia, the frantic promise to wake up becoming so. But coming off sedation is treacherous. Jackie was agitated with the slightest reduction in sedation. In other words, waking up, even barely, and finding oneself in this predicament causes the mind and the body to panic and panic causes those precious vital signs to go wacky, jeopardizing progress and safety.

"Tomorrow," they said, but then again with the reduction of sedation, again agitation jeopardized progress and safety. Another tomorrow of waiting for Jackie and her

It made me cry. One day, Jackie would walk up to them and thank them herself. It still makes me cry.

Though Jackie was in poor condition, her brother described her as "that little champion, still going," each day slightly better than the previous. Jackie received multiple blood transfusions and blood platelet transfusions. Thankful we were for blood donors and blood platelet donors, more rare. All the transfusions and intravenous medications created swelling, ears lost in the swelling. Frightening it was but then we learned, "To get well, you have to swell."   In time, ECMO would go, the infection would go, the excess fluid would go.

One-nurse days, still sometimes two or three-nurse days at a constant pace kept Jackie on track, the relationship between this very ill patient and these very skilled nurses saving our daughter. There were numbers to monitor and tubes to adjust. Some of those tubes, like the ECMO lines and chest tubes, seemed more like garden hoses, attached to machines that pumped in that which was life-giving and pumped out that which was life-threatening: bags of intravenous fluids going in, chambers collecting drainage coming out, wound vacuums, and what all this meant, the hard part, was left up to them.

We had quiet, quiet days and quiet nights, procedures and prayers that Jackie would respond. My son called me a poet for the updates I wrote each night to our online group, our group that grew exponentially. My friend, Kalli, who is a poet, says we are all poets. I wrote without caring what kind of writer I was.

It was the following Saturday, but for Jackie, it was a procedure day and I ached at the thought. Procedures benefitted her, I reeled through my mind. Back to the operating room, attempts to slow down internal bleeding, opening up the chest cavity again, irrigating and cauterizing. More days were big days. Surgeries, doable, necessary, the line we walked over and again. They'd also take a look at her intestines splayed open under rocket-science bandaging as we flew tossed about in this alter-universe. Unthinkably, in the middle of the bilateral lung transplant, Jackie had endured intestinal surgery. So many stories.

What would she say when she learned, the night of the transplant, eight hours in, a trauma surgeon thrust upon us yet another emergency, yet another need for consent, this time for Dr. Erik Teicher to open Jackie's swelling, destabilizing gut? Intestinal surgery in the middle of a lung transplant? "You'll kill her!" I shrieked and gave a ninety-second health history of her cystic fibrosis gut. "If I don't hurry, your daughter will die!" "You're scaring me!" I shrieked as I signed and he hurried away. A swelling of blood, a hematoma, had launched behind her intestines and put her in peril but he calmed it down, good news inside of bad news again.

In those two hours of trauma surgeon transplant interruption, I took the white flannel hospital blanket and covered my whole body and head, a mummied statue waiting. After a long while, rearranging and peering out, there too were my sister, husband, and son, each as me white domes of cotton bedding, each waiting in the same protected worlds. We each peered out as Dr. Teicher came back reporting the news that his intervention had worked.

That seemed so long ago as new forms of crazy-busy swept in, concerted efforts in this extraordinary room, attempts to gradually bring Jackie off life supports. There wasn't room in this room for a mom most days, kind of like there's not room in a marriage for three. What that looks like, sounds like, feels like doesn't take long to figure out, so I rendered myself to the Family Waiting area. Somehow within those hospital walls and those waiting area walls, the place of story upon story, I found myself alone, others around but still alone, and thankfully. Hospitals are places where thinking is heavy and patience is light and I needed to be alone. I'll always remember my friend, Susan, saying I spent the time in Family Waiting willing our daughter to live. No time for crying, no time for begging, willing Jackie to live.

In all of this, Jackie's dad ended up in the hospital with pneumonia. Being up all night more than once over Jackie, sheer-willing people to save his child caused his own resistance to crash. I was caught between two hospital rooms helping manage his care, being present for Jackie, and managing my own mind so it wouldn't start misfiring. Jackie's dad uses a wheel chair due to a rare form of muscular dystrophy that slowly put him there. He spent one week in the hospital two floors up from Jackie, and then he was out. We didn't want Jackie to ever know, our collective secret I knew we could keep.

Jackie's dad and her brother are both named Byron. It was one of those last minute decisions to name the newborn, Byron, and to avoid confusion, we sometimes call the older "Daddy Byron" and the younger, "Little Byron," a name he surely outgrew. Calling them "Jackie's dad" and "Jackie's brother" helped remind me for the time the most important role they were playing.

Earlier in spring with this huge bind nowhere in sight, our plain and bare yard came into focus. Jennifer, who has an enchanting yard in the town of Clifton just down the way, began introducing me to those hardy plants that endure neglect, gentle garden care meandered along until we were gripped by a world far from those innocent by-standers. At the front porch post, à la beautiful porches of Clifton, I had planted a wisteria "stick," leaves sheared off from pulling up surprisingly stubborn roots, found in an abandoned yard across the street among poison ivy, that invasive imposter! Gowns and gloves, both required going into Jackie's hospital room, didn't mix well with poison ivy.

Her dad had said to either water the wisteria "stick" or pull it up, not enough root had taken hold. Any plant in our yard had to be tough enough and strong enough, like we had to be tough enough and strong enough. And I'd talk to the weeds taking over when I'd chance to notice them, tell them to go ahead, opportunistic buggers, just keep away from that hospital. No "weeds" in that hospital.

Among all those crazy weeds finally running amock across the front of our house and those crazy "weeds" thankfully kept away from that hospital room, I soon realized the wisteria stick was full of young pops of verde, beginning to thrive as Jackie was beginning to thrive. She was responding to all of the elements that bring life to a young girl in an ICU. Who cared about those weeds in the yard? My friends would pick them. They said they would.

Jackie's doctors, and significantly Dr. Shalika Katugaha, were winning the battle to eradicate that rarest of fungal infections a specialized DNA laboratory in California finally and fully identified. "Dr. K," an infectious disease specialist, understands the behaviour of pathogens to combat them and apparently she is good at it.

More than two weeks had passed and Jackie was still not awake, still not aware but beginning again to look like herself. I began telling those caring for her about her, that she had graduated from college in Finance in four years in spite of medical interruptions. She worked at Lidl USA, the German grocery coming to the United States, headquartered in Crystal City, adjacent to D.C., urban, residential and commercial with high-rise buildings and underground shops, high-spirited and industrious like Jackie. Her company, too, was high-spirited and industrious, an adventure Happy Jack style. The store's logo, easily recognized, Happy Lidl style.

CHAPTER TWO

WE MADE IT
INTO JULY

The first of July was slammed. At some point, I don't
know when, Jackie returned to the operating room and they
closed her gaping gut. They had left it open to accommodate the swelling and protected it with I don't know what
but the time came to stitch it back and they did. Everything
was in its own time, everything according to their time.

Then one afternoon, Jackie moved off ECMO, which
allowed her to depend more on herself. Still intubated so
unable to talk, still sedated so unawake to talk anyway, yet
I was in her room, assuring her in a one-way conversation
that her life was still there and we were still there. The next
morning, I came out of the elevator and unexpectedly noticed eager caretakers rolling a patient down the hallway.
That little wide-eyed doll peering around from the stretcher
was Jackie heading down for a scan of her new lungs.

They had successfully tapered down the sedation in the
night. Back in the blessed room, groggy and motionless,

Jackie began to communicate understanding "yes" blinks. Blink, "yes" she was in an ICU. Blink, "yes" she had a lung transplant. Blink, she recognized her mother, blink she understood what we were saying, no blink, no she was not in pain.

All of this waking up and "going under" was part of the dance toward recovery, that interplay between sedation and agitation and now also ventilation. All these days after that shocking initial intubation, breathing by way of machine, the time came to gradually reduce that dependency, for Jackie to gradually begin breathing on her own. If too agitated, sedation had to go up. If well oxygenated, ventilation was able to come down. Up, down, up, up less, down more, eventually off sedation, eventually off ventilation, eventually the breathing tube would be out of her mouth and our two-way conversations would finally begin. In this place, no warning, no waiting, they did what they needed to do, when they needed to do it. The dance was complex but they knew the steps well.

Of course, the roller coaster had to start rolling again. Was this a kiddy roller coaster? Some bleeding in her gut caused another fine doctor to take her down to the operating room for another sedation to nip away a small ulcer. How strange to be throttled by news after news, to put trust again and again in these strangers we loved, to depend on them moment by moment, but here we were as Jackie improved in increments. We hoped for no more roller coasters but for boring weeks, weeks being necessary. We were somewhere else far away, unreal but real.

I could never have imagined the potholes and speed bumps encountered taking care of a patient in an ICU. They were steering Jackie's life. That's how my favorite male night nurse described it. He may well have been the genius in the bunch, funny and compassionate. I developed a deep appreciation for him, told him to please let his mother know she deserved the credit. She loved that, as it turned out.

I watched as Jeremy rearranged and replaced IV lines, keeping them healthy and functional, and asked him questions about how they ultimately remove the ventilator. It's the same, he said, riding around that mountainside both hands on the wheel, eyes on the road. We couldn't assume things would be easy. I couldn't assume there would always be room in that room for a mother rocking her girl in her mind, not in her arms. Jackie was cruising along slowly and she looked like Jackie and blinked to communicate. The "tube" would be out of her mouth one day and we would begin a new ride.

I began to write more than updates.

In Out

~~~~~~~~

There's a strange but familiar phenomenon that takes place when entering a hospital. After a surprisingly short period of time, the world inside the hospital becomes normal. Would I exaggerate to say more like the universe inside the hospital becomes normal? Forgive any self-absorption. Conversely, the outside world becomes strange. I slip out briefly to the bank, have to remind myself how to act and what to say. All I want to do is hurry. Get me out of this strange place or at least this strange sensation, I am thinking. Get me back to the hospital.

Our term for this is "in." So if I text a friend whose child also has cystic fibrosis, one word: "in," and my friend knows. And when leaving, discharging, "out." It's an acclimate-reacclimate thing going on even if the hospital stays are not so frequent. It's easy to know. I visualize the opposite of this hospital business being something like heading to Lake Tahoe, leaving one world, entering another world for a while, then back again. This is probably the draw to Tahoe, the feel-good verses the feel-bad of a hospital.

What will Jackie's "out" be like? It will be like no "out" I'd witnessed or experienced. What will it be like for Jackie? I ask every day and imagine it will be phenomenal. The phenomenal will be phenomenal.

Jackie was awake more with facial expressions and blinking, responding well to sedation tapering, wibble-wobbling between less of the medication, then more, then less and less as she could tolerate it. They gave her yet another medication to deal with the agitation due to the intubation. Having that breathing tube inserted in her mouth running down into her airway while awake was freaky and would never become not freaky, but Jackie would live with it rather than die without it.

I wanted to go into that hospital one morning and find that magical wand removed. Not yet. I wanted to find those chest tubes removed. Not yet. Those garden hose tubes out of each side of her chest were still draining excess fluid from her chest cavity into that measuring contraption on the floor and one day I would come in and they, too, would be gone. Progress is anything but predictable in an ICU. I had to accept it.

We were more and more able to communicate with Jackie in spite of the tube of all tubes, the breathing tube. Was she in pain, was her head comfortable, something else I didn't remember since she raised her eyebrows so high and opened her obstructed mouth so wide and shut them down so tight, I thought, "On no! She's annoyed with me!" The nurse thought she was exercising a sense of humor. I knew she was annoyed with me as I had been rattling those questions off like a woodpecker to a tree.

To create a bearable climate, we played a music compilation coming to Blake Shelton's "God Gave Me You." I thought, this could be our little theme song for the day and then I thought, "Oh no!" again. "When she gets 'out' and finds that her mother made 'God Gave Me You' as our theme song, she's really going to be annoyed with me!" Maybe not. What was sure to me was that Jackie would be getting out. What was also sure, Jackie would remain in and out of sedation and we would remain patient.

Dr. Charles Murphy ran the ICUs in that part of the hospital so he was on one ICU floor or another each day, still seeing us often. He was the older guy who orchestrated the ECMO logistics that saved Jackie until Jackie's old lungs could be scraped away and new lungs put in place. He knew we were tough and compliant and impressive. He told us so. He was encouraging when it was hard. Hard was rough but had its rewards and he reminded us of that. We were on the same side, intense and raw.

Jackie's friend Ashley organized meals through a nifty online meal organizing site and probably a hundred meals, everything from store-bought lasagna to gourmet dishes and wine snuck in. Family, friends, acquaintances, and meals showed up in Family Waiting and we needed it all and appreciated it all. Sometimes, we met just outside the front door by the fountain, the door Jackie had entered, the one she would leave by. I'll never forget both Carmen and Amber meeting me there, lips quivering, near holding our breath until Jackie would make it. Meeting by the fountain meant exchanging hopes.

Ashley was Jose's daughter, soccer coach Jose who loved Jackie as we did. Once in the last part of high school, Ashley and Jackie went to a party, guys just out of high school, parents not home. Skipping over the details, by 2 a.m., Ashley ended up in Jose's car; Jose and I ended up at their front door to retrieve Jackie. She wasn't there, they promised. They hardly knew her. Jackie had left through the back gate.

Jose not believing them, wanted to call the police to rescue Jackie but I knew Jackie had rescued herself, her breakaway dry run at breaking away, one of her first attempts at being on her own and I knew it and was okay with it. We left those boys alone and went home and Jackie returned home the next day and that was the end of it. She was on no slope down, knew how to turn it around, knew what she wanted in life. Ashley shared their friendship experience in the letter Jackie wrote to her donor's mom.

> "I met Jackie when I was twelve years old when she was randomly assigned to my soccer team. At first I thought, 'Who is this wild child?' She had so much energy, it was almost annoying. I remember the day we became friends. We were hosting a soccer party at my house and all the girls on the team were downstairs while the parents were upstairs, with the exception of Jackie. It felt wrong so I went upstairs to talk to her and started a friendship that

grew into family. Jackie is my only friend brave enough to tell me like it is and kind enough to want the best for me the same way my parents do. She will tell me if a boyfriend is no good, demand I ask for a raise at work because she knows my worth and refuses to ever let me settle. People like Jackie help the ordinary see all the extra out there in the world. She has taught me to value myself and live every day to the fullest. She may be a control freak, but it's only because she knows exactly what she wants out of life and isn't afraid to go after it."

The Fourth of July was rainy, hopes of batting off the rain, hopes of batting off medication issues associated with pain and double lung transplants, hopes of regaining strength. I wondered if I had developed the same facial expression as our thirteen-year-old shih-tzu, that look like this current world was a bit over my head but if I cocked my head this way and back, if I watched good and hard, somehow it would come to me.

Jackie was awake in increments, able by grimace to express displeasure over the bind she was in. Being intubated flat on her back under a warming blanket, blinking eyes and raising eyebrows was beneath her mental faculty. In other words, she was aware and weaning off the ventilator, but getting out of the bind was tedious work. She shifted ever so slightly and slept some at night, still in the crazy zone, a place unimaginable not long before, unimaginable how grateful we were that there was a way back.

On our social media group, our by-then solid connection to the outside world, were messages about joyous new lungs that made me see the ICU as a place for celebration.

Patients in and out of amnesia-inducing medications need daily reminders they have new lungs, the news of new lungs new to them each day until the news finally sticks. In other words, understanding that she had a lung transplant took Jackie a while to remember and understand, and celebrate. I felt like I was trying to catch bubbles staying positive, and reminders of joy helped. Jackie said later she visualized the joy of enjoying new lungs. She made plans looking far ahead, which helped her get through each day. I continued to think, to write, and post to our group.

Kidneys

I have come to understand that brains are not the only organs doing a lot of thinking in our lives. Every organ is smart. If these doctors here are smart, these organs are smarter. Jackie is on continuous dialysis. Her kidneys reached a point where they decided to protect themselves, as kidneys do, and they shut down, like looking both ways and not crossing the street when a big old truck is coming. Kidneys are smart like that.

Once Jackie's blood pressure fully stabilizes, she will go from continuous to three-day-a-week dialysis and they'll be able to remove the warming blanket and she'll be able to sit up in a chair, twenty minutes at a time at the start. Continuous kidney dialysis machines are not great regulators of body temperature, so I'm saying a prayer of thanks that our bodies are. We live in very narrow parameters each and every day and don't generally have to think about it because everything inside of us is so darn smart.

Once Jackie's kidneys decide that the road is clear, they will safely cross the street to the other side and keep on going and keep on being mindful. We expect Jackie's kidneys to be okay. They took a hit and we will know in time.

Colleen

I have a close friend from college who at age eighteen had an emergency kidney transplant. She went from well to entering the transplant "brotherhood" as quickly as Jackie did. She's sixty-three now with two grown and thriving daughters and, unbelievably, twin grandchildren from one daughter and twin grandchildren on the way from her other daughter meaning four grandchildren in two swoops. She still asks, "How did that happen?" Oh joy!

Colleen and I have engaged in hours of accumulated conversation about her health travels, and Jackie's. They somehow parallel. I already knew that transplants, like graduating from law school or any other major life endeavor, create stories. And here's one about my friend.

Cleveland Clinic took a close look at her later in life, as once again, that transplanted kidney has certainly been smart. So during that recent Ohio visit, my friend had lunch with the doctor who performed the transplant. My sixty-something-year-old friend, interrupting her work as a business librarian, her time at her water color easel, her time with her beautiful girls and quiet, contemplative husband, met with her eighty-something-year-old doctor, and she learned also, her ninety-something-year-old kidney. The deceased donor was fifty, she found out. And they were all three – the patient, the doctor, and the kidney – doing well.

My friend will need dialysis at some point, three days a week. Best to wait until need be, let that kidney continue to "think" as long as it can. But would in all these years my friend and I ever have thought that we would be on the phone looking forward to Jackie going on dialysis three days a week?

I'll never have the medical fortitude to describe what happened to Jackie's own lungs that first of June, but she was the sickest patient up there with a chance of full recovery. This played in my mind all the time. What really goes on in the way of saving lives would be hard to make up. In the heat of early July, which we hardly noticed being enveloped by that ICU, a setback arose. Jackie went back into the operating room with a thoracic surgeon specializing in laparoscopic surgery, most often cancer, this time not.

Dr. Sandeep Khandhar was called in since he's an expert at sneaking in not to disrupt. He cleaned up those chest walls surrounding those good lungs and removed all that surrounding excess fluid, four liters' worth, leaving four small but sure chest wounds, two on each side of the front, two on each side of the back.

I found him to be humble, too, all about doing what he does and doing it well. People at the top of their game don't have time to act like they are at the top of their game and he did not. I have a fascination for names along with a greater fascination for name spellings. Dr. Khandhar's name, and particularly those well-placed h's, would not be forgotten.

He's an engineer like Jackie's dad and they engaged in wonderful hallway conversation as dad had recovered and returned to working in engineering during the day and visiting Jackie in the evening. Jackie's brother returned to his Neuroscience PhD program at Boston University and avoiding a redress, I remained mindful when writing about organs other than the brain being able to think. Most days by then I was solo, Jackie's mom with Jackie in that hospital.

CHAPTER THREE

JULY LURCHED ON

One day, Jackie cried. She got it. She understood because each day in increments, she was briefly enough off the loopy drugs to allow her lungs the chance to begin weaning off the ventilator. Hard as it was for Jackie to look around so scared and in a fix, she was able to settle herself down. If not, the respiratory rate beeper would alarm and motivate her to do so. Those were rapid response beeps no one liked.

In the evenings, the doctors gave those lungs a chance to rest, fully back on the ventilator. The breathing tube remained, that magical wand, the giver of life. We wanted it out but not until the time was right. "Do no harm." So it stayed in and gave us focus and hope for another day. I stayed with Jackie all waking hours. I couldn't read or knit as my industrious self normally would but we were upset and I only wanted to soothe our girl or think about soothing her, nonstop foot rubs inside those sheepy protective open-toed boots she wore.

My mind wondered and wandered, and I wrote using what I could find in that forbidden room, the nurse's pen and dispensered paper towels. Friction in life takes us places we don't expect to go and each day, thoughts echoed in my mind so I scritch-scratched and later composed, keeping everyone informed, letting everyone in.

Not Knitting

"Never Not Knitting" is a blog and before Jackie's hospitalization, that would be me... never not knitting. Knitting is portable and fits well into this doctor appointment life we've lived. Knitters don't want to be called back yet. Knitting can be so simple or can be challenging. On Floor 2 of Heart and Vascular, simple is challenging so never mind about doing any knitting. I'd rather just sit like most people do in waiting rooms. Some of my knitting friends teach knitting. I do not. I help people with their knitting, anytime, anywhere.

What I say to anyone new is that knitting is about rhythm—slow and steady and even. Not fast, not jerky. With fluid hands come even stitches and eventually a lovely garment. This is what nature does when it's not up to no good, the many rhythms of life and I try to remember that they are for us to imitate. Both Jackie and I tend to be jerky. I should say, Jackie is jerky. She thinks quickly and acts fast. I get her to slow down and she does.

Now we're getting her to slow her breathing down, fluid and rhythmic. She's breathing on her own a lot. There's also a rhythm and flow in Jackie's ICU room, the nurses' movements and my movements. We want her to see it and to feel it. No fighting against it. And that's what I keep telling myself as Jackie's status ebbs and flows. Steady.

Yarn needs to glide through fingers. Haste and tension and unpracticed speed result in tangled messes known to knitters as "yarn barf." Today, the super duper laparoscopic thoracic surgeon snuck in Jackie's chest walls and cleaned, leaving no tangled messes but lovely lungs. While Jackie was gone for the six hours in the operating room, I kept saying, "Please no yarn barf" and there wasn't any. Some unraveling, some reknitting, and a lovely "garment" may we continue to make. We were hit twice today with reminders that we are still on that roller coaster and I came home feeling a bit low. But I then remembered that one of the doctors said he thinks we might be at the top and coming down... and may we glide.

I wrote again.

Read this if you want to know how a lung transplant is supposed to go...

Young with cystic fibrosis, lung functions down
Not down enough for a transplant, could hold there a long time
But if they decline, all pre-transplant pieces in place
Continue life, lungs decline
Go to doctor, decision to "list"
Wait for lungs, get the call
Walk into hospital, prepare to launch

Pop old lungs out, pop new lungs in
Walk the next day, circle around the next week
Go to hotel across the street the next month, go home
within three
Lots of doctor visits, lots of drugs and care
No crowded areas, keep away from germs
Few months out, return to work
In the meantime, exercise and sports
Get life back, pursue dreams

Okay, it's not quite that easy. The pop in/pop out part... that would be ten hours. When lung transplants go well, patients are amazingly up and walking within a couple of days. It's still complicated and hard but it's not supposed to be like falling off a cliff. I can't think about it.

I had never paid any attention before to social media, seeing it as a breach of privacy. I understood the benefits of efficient communication and sharing photos but hadn't lived it until this point. The update group our son had created was filled with multitudes of encouraging words, beautiful and creative pictures from so many places: "go, Jackie, go" etched in the sands of the Pacific Northwest coast; "Prayers for healing at the Western Wall, Jerusalem;" a song dedication by Lou and Martin performing "The Cape" in a bar on Ocracoke Island, North Carolina; a Saint Jude Novena from the gulf coast of Mississippi. The Zagardo family sent a family selfie and message from Illinois, "Sending you all of our love, keep fighting." We could not have known at the time Jackie's elaborate, medication-induced, underwater dreams included them.

The Bramleys sent beautiful photography from Memphis, no need to say Tennessee, everyone knows where Memphis is. They made the long trek to Northern Virginia for a few days to help Jackie's father, sick and upset, bringing life back to him through beautiful meals I was in no shape to prepare. I stayed, instead, with Jackie no matter what. I was not about to leave her.

Some days, Jackie slept all day. "You never know what a day will bring," every day. The doctors played medication dodge ball, jump this one in, jump that one back all a balancing act to protect the new lungs, the kidneys, and skin. And then, at the very top bend in her leg, a stitched-up area from the now-gone ECMO hose once inserted there was looking bad. This time at the bedside, Jackie went under anesthesia again. If the bad area was actually worse, Jackie would return to the operating room.

That deep and broad and heavy bruise was not infected and was lifted out. The area was stitched and attached to a wound vacuum for proper drainage and more-sure healing. Between anesthesia and sheer fatigue, Jackie slept all day. The new lungs were anything but the problem and given long-awaited non-anesthesia days and some diaphragm strengthening, Jackie would be ready to face the tomorrows.

We began to meet with strength days. All along, Jackie had been a rag doll. Pick her arm up, it dropped like a rag doll's. Move her finger, she could not. Her wrists just hung there. She couldn't move anything. For weeks prior, anyone moving Jackie caused the medical alarms to go off, her body systems were so delicate. Being "asleep" for weeks disconnects brain from body but, magnificently, only temporarily. Those connections would return with persistent nudging.

Systems began to work against each other and we wouldn't allow them to. Neuropathic foot pain set in, that prickling, stabbing, burning pain caused from nerve fiber and tissue injury creating pain-signaling confusion corrected by the difficult-to-determine right dose of the right pain reliever. Dr. King told us the body does not like to be put to sleep and some effects like neuropathy may be lasting but manageable. Mostly, all of this seemed hardest on the skin and the muscles.

We reached the day movement was tolerable enough that physical therapy swooped in. It was about strength and range of motion and Jackie moving herself a little at a time. The more she moved, the less she swelled. We were getting our girl back over and again.

Seeing her scared eyes again peering here and there, this way, back over that way, I remembered to tell her again that her life with her new lungs was waiting for her and she would be able to move again. For the time, the focus was on strength, most importantly diaphragm strength. The doctors continued to lower the ventilator settings and the therapists worked on core strength. The diaphragm grew stronger.

After seeing Jackie stuck flat on her back attached to everything, ever so slowly gaining strength, I told myself, "Run. Run because you can run." For Jackie at that point, "Sit. Sit when you can sit." That sweet little rag doll would get past the rag doll phase.

I began to bring in photos, personal belongings to notice, remembrances and distractions, demonstrations to all who entered who Jackie was, where she had been, and where she would be one day. More of Jackie's belongings were allowed in the room. I was allowed in the room more but not during procedures like sterile dressing changes. It was no insult. Hospitals are interesting places, so I wrote.

Hospitals

Hospitals are interesting places. Okay, I know museums and sports stadiums are more interesting. Here, you don't easily run into your doctors and come to realize they have their own byways and elevators so not to stop for unexpected conversation, so not to miss conversation with colleagues in confidential corridors. Heading out of Jackie's room into Family Waiting, sometimes quiet, sometimes noisy with family and extended family all talking at once.

Count on meeting others needing to tell their story—triple bypass, maybe heart transplant husband. Want to listen and can't smoothly leave to get back to maybe-awake-and-needing-you daughter right in the middle of what's happening with their kids at home as their lives seem to be crumbling. Learn to be quiet around here, listen to their stories, not tell ours. Too much energy dispelled.

Listen to the doctors. Leave them to do their work. Head over to the café. Not a good sign when the ladies at the cash register start asking if I work here. Maybe an employee discount is in order. Maybe just once say "yes." The food in the Heart Healthy Café is a bit oily and thinking not olive oily. What to select, it's a judgment call and after a while, the stomach will help decide.

The outdoor gardens and benches are restful but there's a courtyard Healing Garden with one small problem: the vast panel of air conditioning units that create supersonic white noise. The air conditioning engineer forgot to consult with the healing garden landscaper. Pretend it's just white noise, wear ear-plugs, or leave. Somehow, the Healing Garden often remains empty, enjoyed from inside through plate glass windows. But there are lovely gardens elsewhere and upholstered benches and two-seater couches in obscure indoor places. There are ways to be alone in here.

Heading back to the room in CardioVascular ICU, standing at the elevator, pushing the button, doors opening and closing, pushing the button, doors opening and closing again, and again. My brain needs to pause long enough to think. Pay attention and get on that elevator!

The room where Jackie now lives is full, and full of calm today, her pain and discomfort somewhat under control. It's number one of five on the white board list of goals for today: manage her pain. There's a stash of Jackie products on the windowsill: cleanser pads, a comb and hair elastics, reminders to her that she's still Jackie and her world is still there.

I used to say when Jackie was little and we were here, "My child is coming out of this place. She will return to the soccer field and slumber parties. Not everyone's child will. And we are grateful." And now, a reality check.

Jackie used to love being better and discharged and eating at the cafeteria downstairs before going home. Not being able to do so while "in" made it somehow special. I never got that but we always swung by and ate before leaving. This time, the uncovering that my child might not make it out of here, finding out so abruptly created in me an unrecovered central nervous system shakedown.

The folks running the ICU say often patients don't remember anything about the ICU. I hope she does not remember any of the events leading up to the ICU either. I hope she wants to go to the cafeteria upon leaving. No, we won't be stopping by the cafeteria on the way "out" but we will be planning something amazingly special when the time comes. And wish the same for all the people we meet in Family Waiting whose stories they also deserve to tell. And look forward to Jackie telling her story, what she remembers.

I thought, and wrote more.

Hate

I hate the word "hate" yet use it all the time. I hate too many rainy days in a row. I hate my dog taking off from the front yard. I hate fighting weeds in the vegetable garden and I hate eating too much and regretting it later. It would be helpful to engage in the exercise of listing all possible words that could adequately replace this inexact word, hate. Interestingly, "hate" is not an expletive though it serves that same satisfying purpose.

People who use expletives say they are irreplaceable and people who don't use them likely do in their heads, though I know some people don't and I want to give them their due credit. Maybe it would be helpful to engage in a serious exercise of listing all possible words that could adequately replace expletives. But for now, I'm sticking with "hate."

Some people hate hospitals, hate going to the doctor, hate having to get a shot. Fortunately, I don't. Fortunately, Jackie doesn't. We thought we hated intubation but interesting how we can grow not to hate under the right circumstance, though I know for certain that Jackie hates how that tube feels.

I also know Jackie is certain that tube for now is keeping her alive. Some things once hated can also grow to be loved. I used to hate stretching. That wait time during a stretch is boring. Yoga involves way too much stretching and waiting, for example. I'd rather be stiff. But now every day, I'm stretching Jackie... each finger, each toe, thumbs, hands and feet, wrists, palms, arches, heels, arms, legs, joints, sockets, calves, Achilles, neck, you name it. Somehow, stretch and hold is no longer boring. I love stretching...all day is fine with me.

There is one thing that I really do hate though and hate is the right word. I hate that Jackie is in pain. That's how her day ended. All that she's been through is bound to involve pain. And they are doing their best to manage it. It's hard to manage and she is feeling it. She hates it and I hate it. And I hope tomorrow will be better in the hated pain department.

It was free Slurpee day, July 11, 7-Eleven, and Jackie was egan having bouts of more awakeness. We called her Uncle Mark who cried and laughed at the same time across the airwaves, all in celebration as he'd been there at the worst. Having more fun with being "back," hard as it was, Jackie asked me to hold her cell phone in front of her and I thought she wanted to take a picture of herself intubated. I took her shaky hand and voiceless instructions to hit that button on the cell phone.

What we did, I quickly discovered, was send an "I'm back" photo out to all of her friends. Some of them were jet skiing and heard screaming from the dock and rushed over. "Ah! Jackie's back!" I had been told not to share pictures and not understanding what I was doing, I had not shared this picture. Jackie had.

People helping Jackie here had stepped up along the way telling us she would not want to see such pictures of herself and maybe she wouldn't. I asked myself many times, what put our daughter in this place, a place we could never have imagined and Jackie would ask the same. I wanted to tell her and didn't want to show her. What had happened and what was happening? Where was she and would she get better? What were the odds?

Odds

Beating odds is my thing. Loving life is Jackie's thing. Maybe my loving beating odds has helped Jackie love living. She doesn't love beating odds, she just does beat odds. And today may be about just that. I get into the car this morning, smart phone says as every morning now, "27 minutes to Annandale." I drive, and ponder. I could ponder an ICU every hour of every day for the rest of my life and not come up with the cascade of events that have tried to take Jackie away from us. One doctor early on said she had used seven of her nine lives and he doesn't know she began her life in an ICU. So when did this beating odds fetish come on my scene?

I remember when we were in elementary school in one of those cool neighborhoods full of kids, the big boys, my brother and his friends, made up a skateboard club. To belong, you had to start at the top of this one steep hill, push off once good and hard, make it all the way straight down, around the corner and up to the fire hydrant. They knew they were screening out the boys they intended to exclude. I watched the big boys do it and decided to try myself. After I made it, I don't know what happened to the skateboard club. It just wasn't anymore.

Beating odds feels good. It's kind of like playing hooky because it's kind of like getting away with something. They're both kind of fun though beating odds is about being there and playing hooky is about not being there. One's about practicing dealing with it and the other is about practicing avoiding it. One's about checking in, the other's about checking out, stepping up versus stepping back. We're all in this crazy world with Jackie though some odds-beating situations like this one are on a grander and more outrageously terrible scale.

So I walk down that corridor again today, find Jackie to be quiet and still and a bit sallow, and go about the mom business of bringing her comfort. Then around 11 a.m., later than usual and never know why, one doctor after another files in. Trach doc-- hasn't seen her in a week, in awe of how strong her breathing is, might not need a tracheotomy when the breathing tube is removed. Kidney specialist-- may be heading off dialysis—eventually, slowly, kidneys have squeaked out a little urine. Surgeon-- wounds healing nicely with the help of this nifty wound vacuum device to speed up the healing. Pulmonologist— Jackie's been on minimal vent support all night. Instead of so many big things like lung machines, her bed is surrounded more by these little pumps that keep her warm, protect her legs, help wounds heal. Wow! Today is a recovery day.

Jackie moves her hands a tiny bit, her arms a tiny, her legs just a bit. She expresses discomfort... because she's getting better and noticing these things like tubes going down her throat and coming from her chest. She wants up. Tomorrow, they will move her to a bed that becomes a chair, head comes up, feet go down. It will take multiple people to transfer her and that makes me sad, but I remember that Jackie is beating odds. She finally falls asleep around seven and I head to the garage, get into the car, smart phone says, "27 minutes to home." I think I'll sleep better tonight. I think Jackie will feel even better tomorrow. I think Jackie will be back. It will take time.

My sister Anne, a school librarian, during that summer moved in with us to help Jackie's dad due to his muscular dystrophy needs. They kept the home and home office afloat and came up many evenings. I loved how Jackie and her dad simply needed to be together, not talking, not interacting, seriously content just being together. Visitors beyond family were not allowed though they occasionally made their way to the door.

Each day, I was at the hospital by 8 a.m. and returned

home each evening between 8 and 10 p.m. I walked away from my life and would not return to my life until Jackie returned to her life and she knew it. I woke up each morning thinking about Jackie already awake. ICUs, living organisms themselves, seem always awake. Mornings are a rush of energy and activity, running tests and drawing blood to determine procedures or what medications to add or take away to keep the patient stable and keep the ICU stable. We all needed to remain stable.

Whine

Sleep comes in portions for the very sick and hearing about potassium levels, white and red blood counts and fifty things more, enough to make me only sleep in portions but I have to be ready each morning so I release in writing each night what "energy and activity" I can, set aside both anticipation and apprehension allowing night to be night, and sleep. To get Jackie well and on her climb out of the ICU, night had to be night and day become day, thus the new bed with chair position is coming to her room.

Then I find out. Steroids, the enemy-friend, help her lungs progress, cause her to not sleep. Sedatives, the enemy-friend, prevent her lungs from progressing, allow her to sleep. Steroids get her better. Sedatives make us think she is better but not. Steroids win. Up, down. The lights and sounds, buzzers and beepers, coming and going and day is night and night is day cause Jackie to start to frazzle and frenzy, difficult to describe. Keeping Jackie in touch with reality, getting her into a more calm day/night routine, hard. Convincing mom there are signs of progress, hard.

I trust them, I remind myself. I trust them because I have no choice. The people running this place, I trust them even if we did have a choice. How did we even get to this place? Jackie cooperated… with her pulmonologist, with her pre-transplant program designed to help her avoid a transplant, to be there when she needed one but not yet.

A good steward of her education, of her career, of her friendships, as a niece, a cousin, daughter and granddaughter, as Jackie girl getting on with her life, living with a dear friend in a beautiful condo, commuting to an adventuresome job, meeting mom and dad for dinner. She wasn't fully well by then so we were going over to help her with groceries and laundry. She was going to have sinus surgery, a help. But not this. She did not deserve this.

Jackie deserved the "easy" lung transplant. Can I whine, feel sorry for us, be mad, get upset? "Upset" is kind of everywhere, in my nerves and bones, muscles and skin, "upset" in my head and heart. It will find its permanent place, fit in that "upset" place somewhere inside, that place we all have but just got a whole lot bigger in there. My heart has to get out of my throat first, return to where it belongs as things in there sort themselves out, as Jackie's body sorts itself out.

Don't think I'm not thankful. Don't think I forgot that someone died, a young girl whose loved ones mourn her loss, a young girl who lost her life the same week she gave our young girl her life back. Don't think I don't know this is a whole lot harder for Jackie than it will ever be for her mom.

Just like I trust this medical team, just like I trust this frazzle-frenzy stage will end, I trust when I learn that patients can leave happy, with standing ovations and Jackie will too. That far ahead is hard to see so we have to face the day at hand and get over "it's not fair" and get on with the ICU getting Jackie well. I have to be present, to bring comfort. The new bed is in.

Jackie made it into chair position finally by 8 p.m. in that super move-about bed. She was exhausted and required ventilator support and pain medication. Enough for one day. She would dangle tomorrow. I thought as I sat beside Jackie sleeping in her new bed, "Blame the disease." When something is complicated, it's too easy to blame a person. Three words always kept me steady, in my work, marriage, any circle of life. I've always looked deeply at what was really to blame and often not a person. For us, for then, and there… blame the disease.

The next day, dangling began, "dangling" being the medical term for moving to a sitting position off the side of the bed. With the intubation coming from Jackie's mouth, big fat drainage tubes coming from her chest, little skinny IV tubes coming from her arms, kidney dialysis lines coming from her neck, with wounds and wound bandages here and yonder, Jackie thought this was crazy. We spent two full days gearing up for this precarious maneuver and enough people were on alert to help control too-dangly parts when we moved her to the sitting position. That day, we reached a "barely dangle." This barely dangler was also moved from critical condition to serious condition. Dangles and condition downgrades made for happy. Jackie's healing skin made for happy. In this place, skin's a big deal so one day, I wrote about it.

Skin

~~~~~~~~~~

Sometimes, I stop and think about skin. Skin is up there with "odds" in my book, though they perform in different arenas. I love skin. We bang skin, bruise it, cut it, burn it, puncture, scrape, pinch and squeeze it, ignore it, complain about it… exhausting though skin never much is exhausted and never much holds a grudge. I don't particularly care for moles and warts and scars but this is the small stuff, I remind myself. I complain about pimples and rashes but really? Isn't that under-appreciation? What about all that skin is doing in the meantime? It's a barrier to the risky world we live in protecting us top to bottom from constant micro-aggressions. When I snag a hangnail with my teeth, I say, "Stop it! Leave that wonderful protective barrier alone!"

Skin faces the ultimate challenges in an ICU. What skin goes through there is terrible. It's just that surgeries and procedures and stitches and more stitches, bedding sheet rub, hospital tape, needles and lines, hoses and tubes… it all adds up to a lot of battle wounds and it's painful and upsetting. But there are wound specialists who do wound care for a living all day long and they know how to patch and pamper, pad and vacuum wounds, to stay ahead of wounds, to keep the integrity of skin from teetering down the slope. Jackie has a lot of wounds and they are under constant care.

Along with sitting up, Jackie's skin is on the up. She's

slowly healing and her skin is slowly healing. When she leaves the hospital, it will tell her story. If you pay attention in the grocery store line, you can spot someone who has been in the hospital by the battle wounds found on their skin. There's a hospital battle wound look. (Jackie accuses me of exaggerating.) I'm not going to be upset about Jackie's skin. I remind myself like kidneys are smart and diaphragms are tough, skin is resilient. And along with all the other doctors, Jackie also has a plastic surgeon helping her tomorrow. The resilient mind, body, skin, and high spirit of Jackie are going to make it. Still a long way to go.

Progress

Being intubated, that breathing tube running through the middle of the vocal cords in the back of the throat, Jackie, fully alert and aware, continues to use her eyes to communicate. Her nurse further develops the shortish list of yes/no needs to isolate—above the waist, yes/no, below the waist, yes/no? Is it pain? Is it her back, the need to cough, adjust her head? Her body is waking up but still no hand squeezes or major muscle movements, small movements, regaining that brain-muscle connection. Physical therapists say young people get it back fast.

Jackie can hold her head up for twenty minutes at a time and they are working on independent sitting in "the chair position" with some support, then sitting independently off the side of the bed, all in hopes of getting off the ventilator. She participates and cooperates fully. It's about balance. Life is all about balance.

Increase strength to get the tube out, get the tube out to increase strength. The breathing tube, the giver of life, made the way and is in the way. Jackie is comfortable, consolable, peaceful, uncomfortable, upset, restless. Jackie looks like Jackie. They have taken the fluid off for the time and her coloring is good. The pedicure, the reminder of what she did before the admission and what she will do after the discharge, still pretty. Jackie, still pretty.

I often called over to the hospital late at night, "This is Jacqueline Price's mother trying to reach her nurse in the CVICU." I would reach the nurses' station and be transferred to her nurse and always good news when Jackie was able to sleep. We torture enemies in war with sleep deprivation and save lives in an ICU with sleep interruption. Jackie pulled out of critical condition in time to somewhat normalize sleep patterns that would somewhat normalize healing and keeping infection away, somewhat clear her mind in preparing to mobilize. Even still, she was wiped out, one day participating in physical therapy with her head bobbing and eyes closed. I spent most of the rest of that day slipping in my own version of physical therapy stretches. My son said I must have been bored.

I was not bored in Jackie's room focusing solely on getting her well. I was bored out in the hallways so I started to notice name tag job titles like Director of Patient Experience, Case Management Transition Coordinator, Senior Director of Building and Support Services in charge of everything non-clinical, and Simulation Nurse Director who helped people simulate being home again. I enjoyed sneak peeking at nametags and began approaching hospital employees like Man on the Street but rather Mom in the Hallways. I always hurried back, Mom in the Room with Jackie gaining energy, moving more, hurting less, and breathing more on her own.

July 16 was my mother's birthday. She had been gone for three years and all of this may have been too much for her. That day was too much for me. I thought Jackie should move and Jackie thought Jackie should sleep and sleep she did, deep restorative sleep. I tried to move her and she got mad. Her whole body scowled. Then every time I touched her, the respiratory beeper went off, raising her respiratory rate because she was displeased, which was not good for her and not good for me, so I left for the rest of the day. All of this can turn you into someone you don't want to be and I had to get away from myself so I roamed around a shopping strip and then went home.

Jackie's nurse called and put the phone to her ear. I was supposed to tell her where I was and when I was coming back. A bit like old times, me talking to Jackie on the phone but this time there was silence on her end. I went back and such a beautiful night nurse who had helped interpret Jackie's voiceless phone call brought good news, the breathing trials were successful all day. The ventilator had been turned off.

I kept quiet, held Jackie's hand, let her sleep, whispered to the nurse and then, she awoke! Jackie opened her eyes and moved her mouth. "I have to pee!" Her kidneys, almighty, I thought! Next those still and twitchy arms began banging on the sheets! Rap, rap, rap! Almighty again! I remembered a chest tube clamp had been caught up under her and was caught up under her again. Getting that devilish plastic noodge out, Jackie settled back into deep restorative sleep. I went home happy that day. More and more of the updates to our group were happy.

Jackie is...

...breathing more on her own, asking for more vent support,

"Ew, turn that thing off!"

...wanting her hair washed, no-rinse dry shampoo,

"Ew, that shampoo is gross."

...asking for her phone, reading text messages,

"Ew, my eyes are not quite focusing."

...staying awake more during the day,

"Ew, get me out of this bed!"

All without a voice.

Pricille

Jackie got her incredible inside out beautiful nurse again tonight.

Jackie knew it

I knew it

Jackie knew that I knew it

I knew that Jackie knew it

Relax Collapse

Good night.

Thank heaven for Pricille.

All Jackie's life, Kalli, the writer and dear friend, reminded us of the stories of our daily lives and encouraged writing. If we don't capture them in writing, we should at least pause and capture them with moments of appreciation. She reminded Jackie that the story of her life has value. When Jackie was in fourth grade, she got permission to spend the day with Kalli doing poetry presentations for the students at Jackie's school. Kalli offered during a break to go down to brother Byron's sixth grade class for an extra short extra presentation. His young, too serious teacher had agreed, "Ten minutes."

Just before knocking on the uninviting door, Kalli realized the props for the poem, "Funeral in the Bathroom," about a class goldfish that had died, these toilet bowl hand-held pencil sharpeners for props were missing. Jackie ran down the hallway and got them. Kalli knocked and the teacher answered as Jackie ran back, the toilet bowl pencil sharpeners spilling from her hands across the threshold. The teacher stared as Jackie scrambled to pick them up. Kalli and Jackie, the writing and the props, and that six-grade class had their ten-minute playful break. Kalli and Jackie were fellow fun-junkies in spite of people who were not and in spite of what may come.

NICU/ICU

When Jackie was born, she was in a Neonatal ICU.

She was born in critical condition associated with her intestines associated with her cystic fibrosis.

She was as sick as a newborn could be.

Her primary nurse said she was the sickest baby she
saw make it out of that ICU.

Jackie was there for weeks.

It took her a while to begin to interact with her
world.

Jackie was determined to live.

That was twenty-five years ago.

Now, Jackie is in a Cardiovascular ICU in critical
condition

Associated with her lungs associated with her cystic
fibrosis.

Again, there for weeks as sick as a person can be

Again making it out of that ICU.

Today, Jackie breathed on her own.

Her kidneys improved.

Her IV medications reduced.

Her infection went away.

Her incisions are healing.

Her hands squeezed.

She makes her wishes be known.

Today, she interacted with her world.

Jackie is determined to live.

This is now. Wow.

Prior to birth, Jackie's intestines developed a blockage
and perforated without warning due to a sticky mucus plug
caused by cystic fibrosis. This recessive gene had not yet been
identified; the tracing was not yet possible. Jackie's condi-

tion in utero was grave and her delivery was an emergency. She was stabilized over her first six hours, operated on over her second six hours. Half-way through, they thought she would not make it but then she did. Her condition became surmountable unlike the newborn with a heart condition next to Jackie whose condition was insurmountable. This opened my eyes and deepened my appreciation.

Jackie remained one week on an open table with heat lights above and tubes all around and a nurse at her side, then in an incubator for two months. I would get up in the night and drive there, call security to escort me through the abandoned parking lot. The NICU was quietly rocking all night long and her nurse, often rocking Jackie who did make it out of there. When we first brought Jackie over the threshold of our home, her father stopped and made me promise, made us promise together not to ruin her, not to treat her any differently than any child we would love and through her childhood, we did not.

Jackie went to college a day early. She was hospitalized during orientation so she had to go early and when we arrived, we saw dozens of large castered canvas bins for moving belongings from car to dorm room. The place was empty except the bins and enough people to help. Jackie would have her space in that dorm in good order in short order and without the bustle and stress of the coming day and the incoming mass of students.

It would have been perfect except she was stressed anyway and began taking it out on her parents. I told her we could take all of her belongings out of the van and drop them at the curb and drive away if she did not get herself together. And we would have. And she knew. And she did get herself together. And we had a delightful day. Little did we know we would go from the raising-your-kid stage to the helping-your-kid-move stage throughout college and after, finally landing at Alyssa's near the Mosaic District, a mixed-use urban concept on the D.C. subway line.

The Beach

Alyssa, Jackie's roommate who owns the condo they lived in, has kept Jackie's bedroom in place and welcomes me there any time. Not that I don't want to go, I can't leave Jackie's ICU life or face her before-ICU life with any sense of ease. Even the thought of finding everything Jackie there except Jackie leaves me breathless. I go anyway. A "Save the Date" postcard designed by "Wedding Paper Divas" addressed to Jackie, "10.29.16 Fredericksburg, Virginia," waits on the table causing a long look ahead. July, August, September, probably not.

My mind drifts as I drift towards the refrigerator, nebulizer medications for cystic fibrosis lungs Jackie no longer has and then a bump, bump, bump from upstairs. Kids. Bump, bump, bump like Jackie's hand to pillow seeking our attention, expressing frustration. My eyes catch sight of the mail order purchase, bathing suits I'm counting on her one day wearing. The "Smith Mountain Lake" beer cozy, I'm counting on her not using. How many bathing suits does one girl need?

This third week in July is beach week. The island of Ocracoke is booked solid, someone in line grabbed our cancellation. We apparently did not need reservation insurance but from now on, we will be getting it. Jackie only got part of that week off but she didn't mind. She loves her work as much as she loves the ocean. She was content with a half-week of beach vacation which has turned now into a no-week beach vacation.

It is painful missing the beach. It is painful being in Jackie's apartment without her, but not as painful as the thought of Jackie never coming back, driving from work blue-toothing with her dad about work, swiping to enter the parking garage, walking down the well-lighted corridor, unlocking the ornery door knob, checking her mail, cleaning up her room, swapping stories with Alyssa about their day.

Alyssa helped Jackie with her care and with preparing for the beach. We aren't at the beach but happy for everybody who is, glad the beach is still there, glad Jackie is still here, not in the condo but not far away yet penned up in that hospital. I get into the car to return to the hospital, turn on the radio, "… Health insurance for people who love God and want to share each other's health bills." "I don't think so," I say out loud. And then Jackie's own writing comes to me. I find the poem she wrote back in high school English class.

> *Beautiful Beaches…*
> *Sitting on the soft white sand*
> *Letting it bury my hand.*
> *Watching big waves crash*
> *Making a big splash.*
> *Seeing kites in the sky*
> *All the way up high.*

Tanning out in the sun
Oh, that is so much fun.
Collecting seashells on the beach
Trying to get each.
Wind swaying in my hair
So it gets a little flair.
Dolphins quickly swimming by
I don't want them to say good-bye.
Beautiful sunsets in the night
They look just right.
Cold water on my toes
They almost froze.
All of this at the Outer Banks
All of this quite nice thanks.

Back in our reality, Lori from my high school who followed Jackie's story and was a nurse asked about our health insurance coverage and I wanted everyone to know that BlueCross/BlueShield was doing their part.

Health Insurance

I was a teacher because schools are fun places to work and students are fun people to work with. The more difficult they were, the more I enjoyed them. A challenge, wrapped my head around it, figured it out, where the "paycheck" got earned. The key to discipline, respect for every single one of them, high regard no matter where they came from, no matter what they had done. I focused, we focused, on where they were going. And at retirement, no more burned out than the day I began (may be a little bit of euphoric recall going on here). I worked gladly and we needed good health insurance, peace of mind.

My friend, Susan, whose son has cystic fibrosis also worked in a school. When she did not and tried to get health insurance, she was told, "We don't insure burning buildings." That was then and we did what we had to do. At that point, the life expectancy of someone with cystic fibrosis was eighteen years old. Now it is late thirties and beyond. Every year as Jackie grew up, her life expectancy went up a year. Good math! Jackie is still on our health insurance plan, until age 26 in one year but we'll figure that out too, always looking down the road.

Right now, we have the best health insurance this country has to offer and it will come through. I left teaching when able without penalty to better help our family though the teacher retirement is being snipped away, health insurance cost increases. But we have it and it's good. We're BlueCross/BlueShield's ambassadors, worth more to them than any advertising plan (always wanted to be good at posturing). We don't expect a financial freefall.

When I signed up, I did not know about cystic fibrosis except that it was something. Our insurance company did know and this is what they signed up for. Jackie might have gone a long time without needing a transplant but that was not to be. They authorized Jackie's emergency double lung transplant. All the right pieces were in place. They've been kind to us. Many bills are paid, all doctor charges, some bills are pending, no hospital or ICU or transplant charges are showing and won't until discharge, as I under-

stand. We are testing the system and know our health
insurance will come through.

We had always tested the system. With Jackie's dad working for himself as a structural engineer, I returned to work
as a teacher. Even a preschooler needs health insurance and
this preschooler, even then, tested the system. Going back
to work was like throwing a cat into a pond. I wanted out
of working before I got there. But when I got there, I loved
it and Jackie loved preschool. She ran like the wind into
University View Daycare and asked me to come back later
when picking her up. Once Miss Margie asked me if she
could take Jackie's meal away, served family style, if Jackie
kept getting up during the meal. Jackie had wanted to play,
eat, play, eat. One time, just once they removed her plate
from the table and she never got up again during lunch. Eat
and then play made for better-happy days. She got it.

In the depths of the ICU, Jackie had better-mad days.
She was getting it. She had been very sick and she was getting well. Time, I told her. She yanked her head left and
right, furiously jerking that intubation contraption in her
mouth. I didn't panic. I simply said, "Jackie, see that nurse
over there. When you were very sick, she saved your life.
She's highly skilled and she worked hard for you. Now you
are going to listen to her today. Do you hear me?"

Jackie's nurse that day was fun sharing grandmother stories with us. Ramar was also tough and strong and fearless.
With grace and ease, she took on the hardest of lives to save.
When she retires to spend more time with her grandchildren, what a gain for them and a loss for us, the ICU folks.
They planned to take the tube out soon and didn't need any
jerky action to screw it up.

Katie

How many –opathies and –osis are there? Jackie's total body pain the other night, ICU neuropathy, nerve endings on edge, an ICU syndrome addressed with medication we don't want but need temporarily, an ICU fix. There's actually an -osis called ICU psychosis, which is either too hard to describe, or too terrible. I may have found the words to describe it and I did find the words to thank God Jackie avoided it. Basically, it's that trick-or-treat scream mask turned ICU horror flick.

A human being, otherwise known as an ICU patient, who has gone long enough with night being day and day being night and neither being neither, adding in buzzers and beepers, the tattle tellers that keep you alive going off around the clock eventually cause this wild scary hallucinogenic ride called ICU psychosis. In other words, the mind and the body are so done with all of it, they rebel, the scream mask turned horror flick.

One tireless ICU psychosis averter saw it coming. She rearranged I don't know what, everything, and it took every minute of every twelve hours of, I think, her three days in there with Jackie to make sane, night night, day day sane.

I thank the nurse who saved Jackie from ICU psychosis and so this poem is dedicated to her.

Nurse
mixologist
tubing
tape
connector
cap, snap, trap
MacGyver
skin care specialist
personal trainer
foot splinter
documentarian
meds regulator
sedentary not
buzzer beater
blood extractor
needler
provisioner
scheduler
traffic controller
implementer
pragmatician
constant communicator
opathy osis averter
angel of life
deserver of thanks
Katie

Jackie would be getting a tracheotomy, a ventilator access in the neck freeing up her mouth though not her vocal cords. She would better be able to mouthe words and in time, eat food. TPN, total parenteral nutrition, intravenous liquid in a bag hanging on a pole with a tube running down into a needle into a vein as a way of "eating" needed to go. Google has spell check for tracheotomy but not for parenteral, nutrition no parent hopes for.

This neat little "trach" contraption allowed the doctors to regulate the ventilator settings like with intubation but also to turn them completely off and back on again, working toward and testing breathing independence. Scaling back using the trach was prudent, rather than removing ventilation altogether by pulling the breathing tube and then needing it back in if the breathing didn't go so well. Shoving a tube down anyone's throat twice in one hospital stay was definitely not good. I could never have imagined a trach could be good but our special nurse said it was and we believed her.

I couldn't believe the swimming pools were open, the daily news continued on, or televisions even existed. I scribbled more.

Trust

How many times do I have to drive into this hospital parking lot and find the flags flying at half-staff? It has to do with shootings. I don't want to know. Would Jackie want to know? What has she missed in the past blur of six weeks? Her world is a box in a box in a box... a bed in a room in a building. Who's in Jackie's room and how many tells a lot. Jackie is down to a half nurse, shared with another patient.

Still, things get wonky in there, daily dilemmas, quagmires always somehow resolved. Life in the ICU is tentative, the ICU, the Tentative Unit. Tentative, "not certain, not fixed," the opposite of "sure and definite." Not in there for no reason and I begin to wonder when Jackie will move out to a less intense unit. Like most of what happens, I will walk in one day and find out.

Decisions and advancements happen when called for, that's when. The intensivist, Dr. King, who saved Jackie's life shows up. I thought he must have been at the beach because he wasn't there for a while. Maybe not needing him as much is a good sign. He tweaks this, adjusts that, small stuff, I wish, but nothing in here is small stuff.

Each day, I wear the only jewelry, a bracelet, a gift from Beth Ann, "Stay Strong." I want Jackie to wear that bracelet one day soon, when she can wear earrings too. I won't wear earrings now because though they take little time to put on, symbolically I don't have time to put them on. I will put on earrings when Jackie can put on earrings. Earrings would irritate me right now like the inability to scratch an itch is irritating to Jackie, or getting that plastic cap she can't reach trapped accidentally under her leg is really irritating to her. Driving Jackie's car, using her water bottle. Not taking that into her room! "Mom, why are you using my water bottle?"

She's that alert and we've learned to communicate in spite of current obstacles. Put on the food channel, maybe not, not for someone who isn't eating by mouth yet. Home decorating is fine for a while then TV off, an irritant. Healing requires quiet. Jackie has found the quiet of night, as well. By seven or eight, I head out of her dark room, her eyes closed, and head home. And call back to the nurse by ten, my eyes blurry. Maybe I can tell by their voices now, the nurturing ones, the ones who will comfort Jackie back to sleep. Should I drive back? I don't. Trust.

Maybe we reached the first day I truly knew Jackie would make it. She was calm and patient, attempting to move about, able to better communicate, and needing me a little less. I was exhausted and tearful, probably an adrenaline let down. Once Jackie could fully communicate, she would so reclaim her recovery and relationships with her doctors and nurses and I would so step back. Her dad also felt more assurance sitting with her that night. His wheelchair fit better in the room. Jackie's garden-hose size chest tubes and drainage containers were removed and IV poles simplified. A new chapter was beginning and we were ready.

CHAPTER FOUR

NOT YET AUGUST

Jackie's dad asked about my writing style. What was going on inside showed up in my writing… and on my face. I imagined looking in the mirror when I got home and finding an old, wrinkled, grey-haired woman staring back. What would Jackie see when she got home? How would she feel after twenty-five years of relentless lung care and then new lungs? Would she run up stairs or empty a packed car with ease? She would be strong and purposeful, very much the same Jackie.

Jackie's Dad Wrote

As many of you know, The Odyssey is about Odysseus' journey home after the ten-year long Trojan War. Coincidentally, I recently have been listening to the audio download. It struck me that Jackie is going through her own odyssey and that she has many trials to undergo before she can return home to her former life and all the people who love her. She, like Odysseus, has various people helping her on her journey home. And her mother is the substitute for Odysseus' patron goddess Athena.

I always wanted to be a goddess. I wasn't feeling so "goddess" right then. Maybe it wasn't all it was cracked up to be. There are many Athenas as any good mother would be. It's what mother would do and happened to be what I was doing until Jackie got her life back. That little goddess actually saw herself on her cell phone. Her shaky little hand, with my help, wrote, "day" to which I told her, "Day 41."

That day, Day 41, Jackie coded. It was a shock. I was in Family Waiting and our tough and strong and fearless nurse was in the room and Jackie had been agitated again. Dr. Brown rushed and got me while Dr. King and his team pulled Jackie back. I stood back from the door both in disbelief and in assurance Jackie would come through and she did.

We never knew what happened exactly, maybe a vasovagal (which is something about dropping blood pressure and fainting from stress), or maybe a hose kinked. I did know Jackie needed to remain calm so not to possibly trigger a need for a code, so I wrote a poster that said, "You have new lungs. You were sick for a few weeks. Your doctors are helping you. You are getting well. We are here for you."

Maybe I should have written, "You had an emergency double lung transplant, were in critical condition, coded a few times, have had dozens of doctors and procedures, remained in a medically induced coma, you are getting back to being yourself and at some point, you will go home, so calm down!" She did calm down. My writing each day did ramp up.

Loopying

Maybe heads-upping happens when stabilizing.

Jackie may possibly be scooting from that unit.

She is no longer antibioticing

And may soon not be tube breathing

But trach breathing,

Unbooting and walking after lots of

REMing and stretching

And forward-looking and believing.

Still carefulling while preparing for tomorrow.

(Loopy mom going to dinner with Lisa, to get un-loopy. Jackie will be horrified one day when she reads this.)

Fickle

Jackie did everything early including going to kindergarten before turning five. At the first quarter conference, her teacher illustrated her classroom personality through a story. From across the room, she witnessed Jackie and others playing house, Jackie being the mom. A little boy bargained to join in. Jackie rendered him the family dog. The teacher found him on the ground begging for scraps at the "dinner table." Everyone seemed happy including "the mom," decisive Jackie who knew what she wanted, anything but fickle.

The nephrologist says that kidneys are fickle, more fickle than smart. I know what "fickle" means but look it up to parse the doctor's meaning. "Change-able" comes first, then "changeful," "inconstant," "as-tatic," "fluid," "checkered." What a word! The dictio-nary even says, "Fate can be fickle like winning the lottery and then losing everything else." How about "losing your lungs and then gaining your life back?" There might be a slight negative connotation to the word "fickle" like the girl deciding not to like the guy anymore but I'll choose to think more like Jackie's kidneys deciding they like her too much to leave her.

Maybe doctors are more fickle, too. The breathing tube is not out of her mouth yet but soon will be. The reason they give: medical prudence. Okay, doctors are more smart than fickle. It's an orchestration and a communication orchestration.

Communication

Maybe it would be easier to be a pet. The whole communication piece would be simplified. If pets do actually make it to heaven, maybe I'm in. Com-munication requires a lot of us, somewhat inex-act, somewhat compromised. The communication among these heavy-duty decision-makers at this hospital seems less compromised. It's as if they've all been in the same training session and came out getting it right, even the shy ones. Did they then go practice in front of a mirror, all of the difficult news they have to launch followed by all of the hard things they have to say?

They told us a while ago they would let us know at any point if they knew Jackie could not make it and they'd have to stop saving her. They had to communicate that. We don't hear that anymore but we do hear not to thank them yet, kind of a superstition ritual around here. I do think I can communicate, "Thank you for saving Jackie's life" but I'll wait.

I am surprised by the intense meetings followed by the flurry of text messaging among doctors to round up opinions and stir communication, to discuss when and how to remove a young girl's breathing tube. Jackie's numbers don't go wacky anymore but when numbers do go wacky around here, doctors appear out of nowhere, effective rapid response communications.

I've been told that there are special rooms in this hospital where people monitor all day long and hit rapid response buttons to the right people. I have a feeling this ICU is one big manning station, everyone on rapid response monitoring, Jackie needing it less and less. Rapid relationship building goes on around here, too, demanding communication partnering between the doctors and all of Jackie's surrogates.

They come in and do their specialty on Jackie, explain, ask, answer, not over or underwhelming. Polite. Clear. And now Jackie will be communicating with them herself thanks to the Blue Rhino Percutaneous Tracheostomy Introducer in the box they just took into Jackie's room. I misread "percutaneous" as "precautious," maybe an inadvertent communication for them to be careful taking the breathing tube out of her mouth and putting this contraption into her neck freeing her mouth at last.

As if there's not enough communication going on in here, there's also the communication from a distance. Hospitals separate people. They create family chasms that no one can do anything about, just tolerate until the time here ends. With Jackie, it has been like communication from a distance while being close, obstructed mouthing of voiceless communications so unnatural, I once naturally leaned my head down and turned my ear towards her. That won't work!

"Jackie. Stop. Relax. Is it your head? Is it above your waist? Is it below your waist?" helping Jackie get away from being uncomfortable and "uncomfortable" isn't the right word either. There's no way to communicate what Jackie's going through.

With her dad here in the evening, their communication has been hand-holding, showing not telling, by the look on Jackie's face. She and her dad have clocked a whole lot of good communication hours over the years and today more assuredly than any day, I know they will many more. I'm thankful for our ability to communicate with our friends and family through all of this, as well. It works. Social media works. And Jackie can now join us. And there will be more communication tomorrow.

Tomorrow

~~~~~~

The breathing tube will be out… tomorrow.

The inflatable leg cuffs to protect against blood clots will be off tomorrow and Jackie be up with the tracheostomy in place. She will soar, still a bit sore… tomorrow.

The Writing

Given the choice between paper and paper towel, I pick paper towel and maybe now always will. Maybe I'll make a run to the office supply superstore and look for the hospital kind. It feels less of a barrier. Rapid scribbles, thoughts to words not lost in the scramble that is the mind.

Maybe it works. Maybe writing works moving the writer into alone comfort. It doesn't take much. Privacy in here comes down to sitting at the café table, the table behind the broad post that somehow does allow the feeling of hiding though the writing itself provides enough. Or sometimes staying in that echoing bathroom feeling bad for the person outside the door knocking and holding it a minute longer.

And then the chair, the hard one in Jackie's room the extra person gets. Take to the corner until tap, tap, tap on a pillow under a sheet. For now, the way of Jackie's shaky rap-tap finger communication. I communicate with the pen. The two come together as Jackie makes her way to her cell phone, to the "Jackie Get Well Update." She scrolls down and my heart shudders, a shudder not found in the quietness of composing but now, what will Jackie think?

She looks and reads and scrolls, reads and stops. She's okay with it but enough for today. Don't fight this. Try to understand it. The writing helps. It makes sense of this nonsensical world, a world we as humans go up against and sometimes we win, where a girl gets what she does not deserve, yet a chance at a life worth writing about.

A Promise Kept

The Associate Director of the Medical-Surgical Intensive Care Unit, Dr. Svetolik Djurkovik, intubated Jackie the early morning of June 13 after fighting hours to avoid doing so. Once he let her know there was no choice, that her heart was playing out, we phoned her pulmonologist, Dr. Williams who from his hotel room far away gave her the confidence to trust this doctor. She agreed but before the medically induced coma, he had to promise she would wake up and he did promise. I don't know how much he meant it, but he did promise.

The Medical Director of Interventional Pulmonology, Dr. Amit Mahajan, and Dr. Bobby, extubated Jackie the late afternoon of July 27. Jackie is slowly moving to the rehabilitation phase. Her vocal cords and surrounding area have to heal so she has no audible voice yet. She is comfortable and contemplative with no memory of what happened, of the promise. She asks,

"Was I listed?"

"How did this happen?"

"What is going on in the world?"

Two Lives

Jackie has two lives here, the one in the bed/soon out of the bed and the one on the wall behind the bed. Once new people like physical therapists start streaming in, time to tape up, with hospital tape of course, pictures of Jackie's other life, the one they don't see but need to see... a picture of Jackie with her Uncle Mark in California, time on the soccer field elbowing her way in front of the girl with the ball, all dressed up to go out with friends one weekend night, her "Wow, that's Jackie?" life.

Other people are leading two lives here, too. Maybe we all do. It's worth stopping to think about. My sister, Anne, moved in this summer to help us, my sister who lost her daughter one year ago by what I believe was a terrible accident, not a suicide. I helped my sister through that and still, she's helping us through this and will. She goes between life right now at our house bridging our gaps, helping Jackie's dad which helps me help Jackie, and her other life, in her home where her daughter is no longer, a home perhaps best left empty right now. She leaves here and goes there, then to work reorganizing the shelving system in her alternative high school library, on to her knitting class, a touch of summer fun in the mix.

And then there's Mo who also helps Jackie's dad, the guy who just spent five years getting his wife here, hurdles with the United States government, hurdles with the Sierra Leone government, paperwork he spent tedious time on. Fatmata, Mo's wife, landed at Dulles Airport last Saturday, relieved and surprised by the number of cars and the kinds of groceries here. Then there's Tabriz, the almost-21-year-old young man I tutored starting in ninth grade, stood by through state testing and assorted growing up near-derailments. I never minded his late night texting about the rules his grandmother set wanting him not to derail. I was just the friend he needed and now Tabriz is just the friend I need, now hired working in dad's home engineering office each afternoon while I am away.

In the late evening, I phone the hospital, "This is Jacqueline Price's mother trying to reach her nurse in the CVICU" in hopes of shedding one life for the other. The one life, the tense street fighter who can't sleep well at night, the worrier of those still-needing-to-wake-up kidneys, the skin that doesn't like tape, the core that can't sit up yet. The other life, the peaceful cooperative helper of nurses, helper of Jackie, the one who knows Jackie will be okay and a good night's sleep will make all of our lives times two work better. And waiting for Jackie to shed one of those lives and pick up her other somewhere far away from a hospital.

The Inn

Late July and still, there is no room at the Inn. The newly placed but broken for-patients-only cushioned recliner cruelly pops up at the head, not down, allowing for only a small puddle of space to curl up and sleep. I sleep in the otherwise quiet Family Waiting area. A tearful woman sits quivering next to a Virginia state police officer, terrible. White-blanketed huddles scattered most everywhere else. Must be a rough Friday night out there. Jackie is having tummy problems sorted out by the twenty-four hour ready-folk but I am not about to leave her and go home.

One ready-folk, a nurse practitioner from a different ICU, shows up outside Jackie's door. People show up from these other ICUs like mystery ICUs in this place. Is ours a "real" ICU? I know it is. She is checking on Jackie's belly that has calmed down so we have time for a 2 a.m. chat about what happened the night of the transplant. I tell her about our white domed flannel sheet all-nighter in Family Waiting and she tells me about the ICU computer access in real time to Jackie's status during surgery. Notes and numbers dropped down into the system and at the hit of a computer keyboard button, these ICU recesses were silently rocking, cheering on Jackie's making it, better than any Super Bowl. The ups and downs had been crazy, the biggest down, prior to the gut trauma surgeon entry. When Jackie came up, they silently went nuts and left for home victorious that morning that feels so long ago.

Jackie's tummy issues resolved, she sleeps well, perhaps the first time in a while in this sleepless joint. Worthwhile for me to be here as "her voice" in this bind and I catch up on sleep once home during her four-hour dialysis session. When I walk in the door in the morning, her dad simply states, "I submit after watching what Jackie has gone through that we think of the verbal representation of courage and fortitude as 'titanium ovaries.'

Over the Week End

A Saturday morning look on the back porch only to find a butterfly adhered to the screen's interior, still, trapped, intermittently flapping, then fluttering about, an occasional frantic somersault. Then, adhered again, still and trapped. Giving it an opportunity to make its way out, I prop open both screen doors. The butterfly will make it out.

By night after a day of helping Jackie cope with being in that room, in that bed, and on that vent, I come home to find the butterfly "resting in peace" across the glass sliding door jam, perfectly formed and motionless, radiant gradient yellows and purples and black. Crap! (another word I hate like "hate") Stop it. It's a butterfly. They start off weak and fragile and stay that way! I pick it up and take it to the far reaches of our fenced-in yard and hoist it over. Get it out of here.

Situations like this invite superstition. That and rituals, some silly external impacting the internal, not likely. Still, in Jackie's room I wash those blue rubber-gloved hands over and again with this special hospital soap we get to use around here, not because those gloves need it but just in case they do. Don't decorate the room too much so Jackie won't mentally leap out of that bed too far too soon, but mostly not to put "overconfidence" in there. We all know how that goes.

Leaving the house Sunday morning, I find another butterfly, this time on the garage door jam, out, free, and happy doing what butterflies are supposed to do. I watch and think, Happy Butterfly. Happy Jackie.

Musings

Good news again. Jackie is switching from intensivists, ICU docs, to hospitalists, the everyday run of the mill docs, the boring ones, wink. As I can tell, hospitalists provide constant continuity of care, their own breed of 24-hour ready-folk in this recovery phase. As I can tell, hospitalists make the doctor life for the rest of them less insane, perhaps altering in time our impression of the medically inadvisable schedules doctors historically keep.

The transplant doctors will still head up Jackie's care because, oh by the way, that's why she's here. She has now shed most all other "side issues." Nothing like redefining the word "understatement," but then many situations do redefine it. Maybe we should come up with some new words to distinguish various levels of "understatement."

A cool new bed request from Jackie is happening these days, "Make the bed longer," "Make the bed shorter." The footboard draws in and out depending on the support the patient needs, mostly associated with avoiding foot drop, that pointed-toe ballet position we all think is so pretty unless stuck in a bed laying flat with covers pressing on the poor feet that want to eventually walk at the 90 degree angle to leg rather than 90 degrees plus another 45, ouch! Those great-idea red-stitched half sheets help, just long enough, not too heavy. This bed capability adds to the cost of this "car" that doesn't go very far.

Not by the bed but by the window, there's a super-sonic forced-air system blowing intermittently. I'm thinking this is one of their efficient ways of "cleaning" the room: suck bad air out, blow good air in by way of some fantastical lever hidden away from view like so many things in this hospital. (Just the imagination going a little crazy in here.)

Time to leave the room for a minute only to walk past the wine cooler, no, the blanket warmer, same look, same concept, warm not cold. Heading out of the ICU, a most unlikely patient appears rolling along on a stretcher looking like she just walked out of the workplace, threw on a gown, jumped on board for a ride down the hallway. Always something to notice, always something to pretend not to notice. Head to Family Waiting. Never thought I would be comfortable rearranging someone else's family room, unspoken protocol when visiting someone's house but here, in spite of the signs to the contrary, the furniture gets moved and we do put our feet on it.

Down to the lobby, where red-coated hosts are scattered about helping people get through this maze of complex carryings on. One asks if I need help getting some place. I start to ask him if he knows where the secret hiding places are around here, just to see if I know more than him by now but I, the thank-you lady, keep quiet and nod and say thank you and move on.

The best form of exercise in the room is dangling, which Jackie is now doing every day. The best form of exercise for the mom is searching the multiple layered parking garage for the parked car I apparently pay no mind to when coming. Find it, get in, satellite radio, turn it on. The news! Screech! The auditory form of tactile defensiveness strikes! Turn it off!

Grab the ten-day parking pass of which there have been too many, remember to turn the headlights on and head home. Tomorrow, maybe I'll notice where the car gets parked. What stays foremost on my mind is what's going on in that room and getting there quickly. The only thing that matters is not hospital musings, but rather "Is Jackie okay?"

It's Hard

What's hard? Lung trials are hard. Being a walking person who can't walk for now is hard. Being a person is hard. It just is. When you're up, you know what's coming, when you're down, you know what's coming, the splashes of life as a person, ebbing and flowing, sometimes waves, hopefully not tidal waves. A wave maybe but please not a tidal wave or at least not again. Before I make a quick switch home, I ask, "Jackie, can I do anything for you?" She responds voiceless in the quiet of her sheets, "Take me home."

The miseditings of my writing that my friend, Lisa, said slowed down as Jackie improved, now creep back in. I think, "Jackie is melting away in those sheets." But deep, honest, and sincere lung trials do cause fatigue and it's hard. How can her lungs improve when her diaphragm is stuck in a bed? I'm tempted to make that first call to her doctor's cell phone but I'll wait.

Head home, walk into my husband's home office,

"Please don't tell me you're not okay!" He is okay.

I head down the opposite hallway past my sister's summer bedroom and notice the small fan blades flying around in their little circles. Turn it off! We don't want a house fire! Give that little blessing-possible cursed fan a rest. Maybe I am engaging in my own musings, mind musings. Maybe mind musings right now are exaggerated due to our child being for weeks one kinked breathing tube away from leaving this world, though not so considering the reliable multi-complex systems in place, numbers and alarms, alarms and numbers. Comes down to more than that but seems the numbers are the truth-tellers and the alarms are the tattle-tellers, both the kind we like.

Easy to start to lose it here but we can't! We've lost enough already, and gained. Jackie, more like it, has lost enough already, and gained. How far can a body go? Jackie's tells us, far. How far can a mind go? Jackie's tells us, far. My mind tells me it works and then plays out some, like maybe right now my mind is playing out.

I head back to my husband before I head back to Jackie. "Sorry about last night." How are those personal coping resources doing, I ask myself? No yelling going on here, thank goodness. Yelling, the indicator of personal coping resource depletion, all the possible strategies either used up or lost somewhere and that's what's left. Fussing, too, as my husband and I were doing last night. We cannot do this. When it's hard, do not turn on each other! This cannot seep into our lives. Reach down deep and find those good personal coping skills making ready the home that Jackie will come home to. We have, we will.

While gone, Jackie's cousin, Josh, is in her room bringing a desperately perfect blast of normalcy. Jackie wakes up, voiceless talking, much catching up, sitting off the side of the bed on her own, making happy her cousin, those helping her, and those passing by the door who know what progress looks like. Some find out before I find out, Jackie's update entry tells everyone, she's alive, awake, herself, visiting with her cousin. And then Jackie says, "I'm tired. It's hard." She sinks back into those sheets. Joshua will come back. Her cousin Christie too, who also brings into the room confidence that Jackie's life is still there. Her brother Byron will be here later in the week. And in time, Jackie will go home. Jackie will be okay. She just has to be.

Time

Time is supposed to "wound all heels and heal all wounds." I've learned that "time sometimes answers some questions and sometimes questions some answers." At times, I learned not to ask. When Jackie was first in "critical condition," I thought, doable. Then I find the American Hospital Association's definition of "critical condition" as "vital signs unstable and not within normal limits, patient may be unconscious, indicators unfavorable," likely not doable. Glad I didn't ask. Jackie moved towards "cautiously optimistic," "serious," "encouraging," "stable," and now I hear something about "home."

The American Hospital Association does not like term combinations like "critical but stable," and though their goal, too, is home, no mention of the word "home" in their online resource guide. I hear Dr. Brown at Jackie's door, "home port" and "home cath." I am not going to ask but wonder if "home" means easier to manage or that Jackie will be going home. Physical therapy helps Jackie sit, not stand yet, and then off to the catheter lab, not too homey.

Upon returning, Dr. Bobby does a bronchoscopy as Jackie watches on the computer screen, the lighted camera going down through the trach opening in her neck for a look. The new lung stitches are beautiful. Glad to see them. Lastly, Jackie has dialysis. I begin thinking, "home" does not mean home. Jackie is Jackie and she has been awake all day, in a good mood and doing well, moving along towards home. Not asking when. By listening and not asking, "home" is really "Hohn," a brand of central venous catheter. I needn't know more.

The day goes so well, I sleep well through the night and wake up to find that Jackie did not. Three am, smacked by pain, all over pain we all know about or maybe we don't. I rush in the etiquette-challenged elevator, the one used by loved ones rushing up to their aimed ICU floor. Elevator etiquette. Maybe we should wear signs in there, "Wait! I need to get out first!" before others dart in like cutting in line at the interstate exit back up, annoyed and wanting to blow the car horn but not because doing so would be silly. Maybe there's an unspoken simultaneous forgiveness as the elevator doors open in this challenging place.

In the room, Jackie reacts to anything I say by the stressed look on her face in spite of clear skin and clear eyes, her pretty Jackie look back again. I think back on teaching days driving to school in the morning challenging myself to discipline the whole day without words. Verbal people like reading teachers, like English teachers, like me, want to cure all ails with words. Silence and stillness, taking a break from helping Jackie with words, gentle actions and gestures, doable like disciplining twenty-five seven-year-olds without words. Best for Jackie right now, best for her recovery.

Everyone in her room focuses on gentle breathing to help Jackie focus on gentle, ventless breathing, breathing on her own. Her new nurse is quiet. As they are quiet with me, I am quiet with them and the opposite, taking thought to allow them to nurse Jackie in their own way, adding into Jackie's day their own personalities. It is more about stepping back at this point, Jackie taking over her own communications. Loving Jackie without words isn't hard. We are ready. She will pick up her pace, and for both of us, it's about balance, and time.

Jackie began just a little updating the social media group herself. She wrote that breathing without the ventilator was hard, staying calm and relaxed was hard. She would stay off as long as she could each day until completely weaning off. This major milestone was still about strengthening muscles. Another major milestone was passing the swallow test, which meant finally sipping juice.

After those initial two hellish weeks of witnessing critical condition and all the trappings, Jackie's brother had to return to school in Boston. I called him one morning and said, "You won't believe what happened?" which broke our careful-with-language rule so as not to alarm him unnecessarily. I was waiting far too long not far from the hospital as I had witnessed some gentleman's tiny little vintage sports car get smashed at the intersection in front of me.

Byron's mind was on what he had witnessed, the thinking, studying, directing, negotiating Jackie out of peril, to head her back towards those fifty pairs of shoes in her closet. Then he had to return to school so he could hardly imagine the progress we were witnessing. He had to come back.

No nightly phone call could prepare her brother. He rushed into that room, throwing himself against that bedrail with tears and disbelief that he got his sister back. Those were two close-to-no-pain days and hours of the comfort of having her brother visit.

Another Stay

It's the weekend again and I have to stay, this big town ICU not like a small town B&B in spite of the accoutrements. The challenges of recovery, the yearning to walk, to get life back, seem like forever, feeling worse before getting better, so I stay. I want to and need to. Jackie doesn't remember the "that was then" part, so "this is now."

Rebellious kidneys seem to be doing a little showing off again, causing swelling. After the sucker punch they took, no need to badmouth them. They are still letting us know. The good kidney doc adds medications to encourage the kidneys to kick in, and takes medications away, pushing them hard and nudging them along. So much to learn, too much to know.

"How does someone walk away from a life helping someone in a hospital?" my son asks. The answer is shared between Jackie and me this weekend. "I'm in hell." "I'm in hell with you, Jackie, and we're going to get out of hell together." We are not really in hell but to insist is to resist and the personal empathy feels right.

Wearing a yellow paper gown and blue rubber gloves, I apparently sleep-walk from the barely-reclining chair to the disposal bin and shed a layer of "hospital." Up off and on all night helping Jackie get comfortable, I need to be comfortable. The first night makes the second night worth sleeping there. Jackie finally sleeps well and during the day, I finally slip out.

Wandering

It's Saturday and I make my way over to Jackie's apartment again, over to the perfumes and creams, mirrors and photos, books and blankets and candles, and shoes. We don't have to pack it all up and send it off to somebody else's life. These are for Jackie's life, real and present and waiting. Soon, we will hear Jackie's voice again so missed making plans with the people she created such a good life with, and the clack of her shoes on the floor, hear her laugh as her thumbs fly across those cell phone keys sending funnies from her dad to entertain friends.

On the way back to 3300 Gallows Road, I cozy up for twenty minutes to the Sweetwater Tavern bar seeking a home brew double IPA deciding not to sit on that misplaced stool behind the beer tap dispenser. No need to hide in this free and easy place and no need to get a little weird. Friendly people are all around but somehow I keep a secret while there, that our daughter lies just around the corner in a situation they would be lucky to know about but are rightfully too busy to. I keep quietly to myself, nudge up close to the bar, and wonder how many people use Sweetwater Tavern as a Fairfax Hospital escape joint.

Walking back in from the hospital garage, I realize at that late hour to buzz in. "This is Jacque...," interrupted. He already knows and the doors open. A phone call comes in the elevator, caller ID, "Jackie." No sound on the other end, not yet, and then a text message alert Jackie-style, "Come back." Those leftover TexMex rolls Jackie can't eat get tucked away. Her first set of plans hatched the previous weekend with her brother, restaurant rounding as soon as she gets out. Glad she has those digital native fingertips to two-way communicate with her brother to keep the plan going.

By Sunday, I glance at the vent screen, "Patient Not Ventilated. STAND BY." We'll stand by all right because standing by means huge progress. Spirits lift, doctors and nurses bring encouragement, good news about progress and plans for more progress, smiling as they talk to the real live and so cool girl getting her life back.

Leaving Jackie became a little easier, especially with a limited number of friends finally visiting. Regretfully, one of those first routes out during the day had to be to renew my expired driver's license.

DMV/ICU

Normally my husband goes along to the Department of Motor Vehicles because the security officer always peers down that long line and sees my husband's wheel chair, which means a go-ahead directly to the service window. I never understood that. The only guy in line not standing, the one with the comfortable seat gets to cut in line? It must be a policy as every security officer is not that wheelchair sensitive.

My husband would advise going over to the Goodwill and getting a wheelchair to use on occasion. Once in DC, he approached a beggar seated at a stone wall outside of a museum. After discussing if he made a hundred dollars a month or a hundred dollars a day, which the guy denied, Byron said he wanted to give that line of work a try. The beggar said, "Oh, you'd do real good in that chair." Byron, from his wheelchair, suggested this guy go over to the Goodwill and get himself a wheelchair to which he said he would never cheat his customers like that.

I get to the DMV by myself, a three-hour wait. I have no choice but to pull the ICU card. Since Jackie will be moving to a rehabilitation hospital at some point, glad I am able to be honest about the ICU though it would cross my mind to pull this after the ICU. The temptation will linger. Cutting to the front of the line is clearly a stress reducer.

If you want to pull the ICU card too, you can. Just do it on the day you come to visit Jackie and let's stretch a little, even if you only make it to Family Waiting outside of the ICU. We only have until sometime in September so check your DMV records and get in there if you need to. When all of this is over and Jackie is home, I wish for her a permanent ICU/DMV card. She's done enough waiting already.

Touch of Dad

Dad, mom, and Jackie are sitting together at the Fairfax Hilton, I mean Hospital, waiting for the bedtime pharmacological cocktail. Jackie ate gelatinous gruel earlier, easy to swallow, bad to taste. Jackie also walked for thirty seconds, three people holding her. There is liability in all of this.

Her dad speaks of the beneficent mechanical Dracula, known as dialysis, swooping in earlier and I speak of the wound nurse praising wound recovery on Jackie's abdominal battlefield map. Swelling causing blistering caused "battlefield mapping." I close the shade to prevent a five a.m. arousal and our communal enterprise ends for the day.

The View

The view from the room, a view in the room, a reminder of why we are here and that we will leave…
Raise the shade before the sun reaches the top of the

sky and pull it down as night falls, feebly imitating in this room life outside of this room. Across the gravel pitchless lower roof rises the adjacent plate glass windows, life in that room, the operating room. The room over there remains quiet and then movement, caps like night caps yet anything but the quiet of night, the surgery ready-makers. The view from Jackie's room is the room that saved Jackie. We watch and we give thanks for that room where shades go down, other lives saved.

I'm assuming they've all taken the Open Chest class, date and place and time posted on the ICU entry door. The class, I learn in fact, for those times when these rooms here across from the operating room become the operating room, the emergency saving lives maneuver, changed quick into one of those. Magnificent. How do they do that?

Taking a view in this room, what is happening to Jackie in pain right now? The Knowingest One, Dr. King, the gracious decision-maker, the one you want when you might die and then get to live, is on transplant rounds and baboom, he explains. It's the anabolic/catabolic balance, of course, the process of building up requiring energy, that of the young and well versus the process of breaking down releasing energy, that of the aged or ill. Life comes down to metabolics.

Jackie's young, anabolic-dominant self allowed her to survive this major medical event and will allow her to get well once the balance tips back. For now, we're holding here anabolic vigilance. Nerve-muscle connections, voice recovery, kidney cooperation. Jackie is complicated. Isn't everybody?

Jackie had to go back on ventilator support, a day of complete rest from lung trials off the vent. It sure felt like going backwards though we were assured she was still moving forward. Thoughts went, to be sure, to the summer missed.

A Summer Missed

Wisteria brown leafed waning
River birch grounded leaves below
Summer heat making a little crazy
Squirrel hanging in hopes persistent
Gold finch seed supply ever-wishing
Empty bird feeder failed summer treat pursuit
Humming bird nectar dormant
Newly butterfly bushes withered
Forget about the summer missed
Curtains closed hundred-degree heat out
Excuse to keep summer out
The summer that wasn't
Jackie cries of disappointment
Summer events gone
Realizing this medical event
Wisteria new shoots spring
Greenie leafed red-berried magnolia thrives
Hope in the hearts of squirrels and birds and us
Autumn forward looking
Making it home

A summer missed

My friend, Sarah's reply, "a gold medal summer" and I thank her for saying that.

Before this tidal wave of a medical event, Jackie was selected as an honoree among young professionals with cystic fibrosis in a 15-week Cystic Fibrosis Foundation summer fund-raising campaign called DC's Finest. I happened to check her phone texts just after her lungs tanked and, "Jackie, just want to make sure you're ready for the kick-off Wednesday night!" Oh no! One of the few things I followed up on those days.

Two weeks before DC's Finest, Jackie attended a local Bobby Bones book signing and shared these words in a follow-up letter to engage him with the fundraising:

"Did you know the average person inhales 28,000 breaths a day without even thinking twice? I, on the other hand, take 28,000 breaths a day and think about every single one because none of them come easy to me. Every breath I've taken over the years has become more and more difficult. Who says you need strong lungs to be happy? I push through every day. I wake up Monday-Friday and go to work as a financial analyst for one of the largest retailers in the world and spend as much time on the weekends as I can enjoying myself with friends and family. Fight. Grind. Repeat. Life doesn't stop for anything and I can either let this disease take over or I can fight it, stay positive and live my life like there's no tomorrow. So I sit here writing this letter (hoping you read it), glad I have that strength..."
Jackie signed, *"Stay Pimpin Joy."*

After Jackie's double lung transplant, her friends sent a blast of emails to Bobby Bones. Who is Bobby Bones? Wikipedia says, "Nationally, The Bobby Bones Show is the biggest country music morning show in the country, with an estimated audience of nearly 3 million listeners. The show's largest market is Washington, DC, where WMZQ airs it weekdays from 6 to 10 am." Bobby Bones sent Jackie a get-well video. It helped. It all helped.

Jackie's ability to engage in her care discussions and decisions grew stronger as her new lungs cooperated. God love that sweet duo! Her voice was recovering from the swelling and nerve injury associated with intubation. She went from "eeking," a speech therapy term, to making audible voice sounds, not words, but sounds.

Tubes

In a way, this place is about tubes, putting things in the body or taking things out with tubes, tube management. I couldn't help noticing the guy next door finally free of that taped mass across his nose anchoring the tube leading down from his nostril to access his stomach to drip nutrition in. No fun. In some countries, they require nutritionally challenged children to thread that tube down nostril to stomach every night and back out again every morning. At some point, tubes are damaging: rubbing up against throats, esophagi, even the inside of veins, and I know this is one more area where these people are careful.

Here in "the States," cystic fibrosis patients get a g-tube, a silicone button valve resting on the skin like a second belly button, with a flip top on the outside and a hollow stem running through a hole to inside the stomach, then anchored by a small water-inflated balloon resting snugly in there to allow nightly hook-up convenience. Those one to two thousand calories slow-pumped in all night long by way of a hanging bag filled with nutritional goodness, canned formula.

Jackie still ate during the day, greatly boosting her caloric intake, greatly boosting her nutritional status, general health, and ability to fight infection, by golly. Who would go through all of that otherwise? Jackie has had one since age eight with an interruption during college when she begged off it since it seemed so freaky at that age.

When she first entered Robinson Secondary School, I watched that tiny brand new seventh grader select one of those sixteen doors running across the entryway and learned later of this story. Drama class, day one, big circle, teacher said, "Tell us something about yourself." The class froze. Jackie didn't. "I have cystic fibrosis and this is what it is... and I have this button on my stomach and this is what it does..." and pulled her shirt up, showed it to them because it stuck out a little, lest someone should ever ask. And finally, "Any questions?"

Turned out, one little girl had a bike hit-and-run short-term memory brain injury and was in recovery phase and another little girl had a "wooden leg" traded out as she grew. Jackie came home from school one day and said, "Mom, Heather's leg fell off in class today and I had to help her get to the bathroom to put it back on." By the end of the year, the drama teacher nominated these three girls who each won an award and there they stood up front to be honored at the Optimist Club dinner celebration. Catch it while you can.

Jackie outgrew that willingness in short order but she never outgrew being too okay with her g-tube, which her dad always called her "internet hook up." So that's how Jackie's gotten her nutrition in the ICU once IV nutrition was discontinued, through the g-tube. Just now, she's imitating mealtime by taking a bite three times a day "by mouth," though interest and taste have not kicked in and eating is tiring, believe it or not. Being someone who lives to eat, I can't imagine but I am witness to Jackie slowly beginning to eat, slowly needing fewer tubes.

Obstacles

Ten o'clock in a thunderstorm, we head out of the house. My husband gives me a look. I tell him that Jackie needs us and we have to go. The back way to the hospital, the route I take every day, that bridge at the bottom of the long dip in the road, is flooded out, indicated by an all lighted up fire engine blocking the way.

We route around and then, the hospital all lighted up by police cars, both getting there and being there blocking our way. The hospital is on lockdown with hourly updates, a disgruntled emergency room goer wielding a knife at the green parking garage decides to end his life by police, well, protecting the rest of us. We'll never know why.

Some questions don't get answered, some do. Why are Jackie's parents there? Jackie is understatedly uncomfortable and her nurse tried her best, so in spite of the terrible mix-ups in the stormy outside, we slip our way into the quiet and still interior. By midnight, with my daily care know-how and that touch of mother, Jackie falls asleep until morning. Her text to her mother before coming that night, "God help me." Mom helps her, thanks be to God.

There are more return nights. One night while the medical team is mitigating the collision course of Jackie's symptoms, I go back and make a tear-filled three-way call along the way. Connie and Cathy are sisters and I met them, like Brian in our group, in middle school. In fact, I met Brian at Cathy's house in middle school. I need them to listen and they do. They do as they always have. The doctors steer Jackie out of whatever obstacle trying to get in their way.

Feeble-handed, jagged and pained non-word scribble on paper turns brief, gnarled, erasable white board messaging and finally, short but effective phone texting. Here are a few text messages from Jackie over these days.

"Come back"

"Hurry up"

"Where are you"

"Please come back"

"Will you fix my hair"

"Will you fix my feet"

"I feel so sick"

"I hate being swollen"

"I'm so uncomfortable"

"I feel like I'm moving backwards"
"God I wish you were here"
"God I wish I was home"
"Mom stop your starting to get annoying"
"Why did you move money from my account"
"I don't like Coke anymore"
"The food lady told me she's praying for me every day"
"I really want a Reuben from Park Ave Café"

The funniest text comes when this very kind old guy comes into Jackie's room to do dialysis. He tells her long drawn-out stories, taking too long for set up and way too long for take down. Jackie texts me with the old guy in the room and me sitting right there or just outside her door. "Stop talking to him." "He'll never finish." "Cut it short, mom." "OMG, this should take ten minutes." Not being able to talk, Jackie can still rule by way of her phone.

Another Funny

The funniest mom friend story was when Jackie was in elementary school. When she was mad at me, she would say I had no friends. "Mom, you have no friends." In fact, I was friends with her two elementary school clinic aides, the ladies who took care to give her pancreatic enzyme capsules before every school lunch, a demand of her sticky mucus disease, sticky mucus blocking up the pancreas and access to her own enzymes, thus the need for enzyme capsules every time she ate and to this day. Capsules hanging around school lunchrooms alarm people so the clinic kept them safe.

I happened to be at dinner with Linda and Margie, enjoying the crawfish special, when I mentioned to them Jackie's favorite revenge. Seeing her every day at lunchtime, they did know this little girl. They called her and placed the cell phone on speaker on the middle of the table in the middle of the restaurant and laughed that they were her mom's friends, that her mom had friends, they were proof she had friends.

Jackie wasn't quite cured of the comment but when she pulled out of her ICU bind, she told me, "Mom, I am never again going to tell you that you have no friends." My friends are now her friends. Her friends are now my friends. I now have some of their coveted cell phone numbers and some of her doctors', too.

Wracked Nerves

Jackie's beautifully dressed, spicy and exotic infectious disease doctor, Dr. Shalika Katugaha's family is from Sri Lanka. "Dr. K" continuously carries the heavy responsibility of what to prescribe in what dosages to combat what infection, and not combat the health of the human body. She explains that pumping super-sick people full of fluids protects the heart, and the swelling known as edema does eventually go down. Not yet.

Swelling is up again and swelling is no fun. Large

ankles and legs, large arms, even wrists, feel terrible for a tiny girl who reaches nearly twice her weight at two hundred pounds. Feels like risky business to us but Dr. K is in the risky business business and executes with seeming unwracked nerves.

Jackie's gently seasoned nephrologist Dr. Andrew Howard, we love him, explains again that kidneys dominate so they let kidneys think they are dominating and sneak behind their back and use medications to assuage them into submission. The kidneys, in the midst of all possible interventions and dialysis support, may begin doing their job again soon and rid the swelling.

A bilateral lung transplant turns into a recovery battle with the kidneys. Dr. Howard was there from the beginning meeting with Dr. King in remote quarters brainstorming the prevention of permanent kidney failure. Along with Dr. Katugaha, Dr. Brown, and the other doctors, they complete this communication circle of medical success. All their hard work and patience, and all the explaining somehow soothes our wracked nerves, wracked nerves reflected in some of the questions Jackie is asking.

"I wonder why I have a tingly feeling up my whole leg now?"

"Do I have anything to worry about and can I see the x-ray of my old lungs?"

"When do you think I will be able to enjoy my new lungs?"

"So do you think the feeling of having a board pushing on my front is ok?"

CHAPTER FIVE

AUGUST BROUGHT SUNSHINE AND SHADOWS

I was sure if I looked up the word "recovery" I would find the definition of "catawampus." Recovery is the process of the body seeking balance and in the meantime, the body is out of balance, askew, awry, catawampus. Recovery takes time, three to five days for every one day being sick-sick. It's demanding and frustrating, amazing and remarkable. These doctors aimed for Jackie to be home in October, six weeks away but between this time and that was catawampus.

Catawampus

A quiet day
A quiet night
Issues come
Issues go
A shooting pain

Blood pressure rise
An eye infection
Shaky hands
Small stuff
ICU stuff
Addressed
This is the place to be.

Resilience

~~~~~~~~

What is resilience? How do we get it? Can we lose it?
Is it something like confidence is something? Sudden
or over time or both? Does anybody really know or
are we still guessing like we're guessing on quick on-
set deadly pneumonia? If there's a book called "Resilience," why read more than the title? I get it. Some
trains we can't get off but with the help of resilience,
keep off that one train, the crazy train, always leaving
the station, always pulling us on. "You can go to the
station but don't get on that crazy train," my husband
always says.

One of the jobs of these people up here is to help
people like us from springing a mental leak journey-
ing through these medical miles. I learned early on
from this insightful doctor about half way through
a hospitalization, at critical mass, we can make it
through without a meltdown by knowing it's coming.
Humor helps. We went through this when Jackie was
born and humor helped. Once standing with a doctor
staring into Jackie's incubator in the Neonatal ICU,

he told me, statistically speaking, our marriage had no chance. I looked at him and gave a gentle laugh but in my mind thought, "Want to bet?" A beating odds challenge. How odd, how funny.

A second time peering in the incubator on the eve of the definitive diagnosis of cystic fibrosis, couldn't feel worse that day, I relayed how my husband and I had determined the inevitable. The earliest writings of cystic fibrosis, infants who tasted salty reported as bewitched and did die. This disease creates a salty taste to the skin. So I unthinkingly told this doctor we already knew, that my husband had licked me the previous night, I had licked him, we kept licking each other and no, we weren't salty and yes, Jackie was salty. Okay, maybe someone else could see it coming but on the eve of one of the worst days of my life, not quite. The doctor's response, "Mmmm!" I looked at him and rolled my eyes but, well, it was funny.

They brought in Pat, still my friend, who brought in a photo album of her son, Danny, still Jackie's friend, letting us know that we would have a life, that we could do this. We have and we can, Jackie has and she can. Maybe we drew the lucky card in mental health, though I'd like to think we've worked it through and will continue to.

Anyone hanging around long enough knows I throw this stuff around in my head. Not looking for a redress from those mental health experts who warn us not to trivialize. We're process thinkers. It's been my survival and Jackie's, definitely Jackie's. Work it through. I imagine she's now at a place few people go and most of the rest of us don't even know.

One of the first moves Jackie made when her fingers started working was to check her bank accounts from her phone, thinking and moving along. So last night I told Jackie I needed to go home early and catch up on missed sleep, didn't want to end up with cytomegalovirus, a possible threat to Jackie's new lungs. She said back, "It's not my fault you're not willing to take the melatonin!" She's back! And Jackie's laugh is back! And they removed the vent from the room. For a short trial, no vent. For the long trial, yes resilience.

Happening Places

Besides the CardioVascular ICU being the happening place, instant resolution zone, the gift shop at the main lobby beats the mall any day if you'd been here long enough. I notice the ladies working the cash registers wearing volunteer pins, their names and hours like "400 hours."   My first thought besides "thank you" is, "I would never have 400 hours to volunteer for anything! Wow!"

As I head down, I hesitate as apparently news hasn't traveled north to the second floor addressing the bathroom labeling issues, still "Men's" and "Women's" single-use arrangement everyone ignores except the vigilant cleaning staff who keep the "Men's" from smelling like "aim and miss."   I prefer the first floor multi-use "Women's" with the huge stall at the end with plenty of room to hang your hat, so to speak, next best thing to going at home.

Heading to my gem of a dining spot, single table behind the large dining hall post, I meet a lady wearing a name tag all spelled out, "Quality Improvement and Outcomes Manager, Quality Regulatory Preparedness," a welcoming facilities management person, yet I forget to ask her about the second floor bathroom labeling.

Returning to Jackie's room, I stop at one of my favorite hiding places, the vacant pay phone booth-like nook at a turn in the hallway just outside of Family Waiting, an unsuspecting place to make that long-awaited private cell phone call. The wood plank of a seat remains, thank goodness, as does the punctured wall where the maintenance worker apparently yanked out the pay phone. Bet that thing has antique value.

Back in Jackie's room, the BlueCross/BlueShield Hospital Coordinator drops off literature and her business card. She was instrumental in the transplant surgery authorization, I find out, and will not miss the opportunity next time to thank her. Our insurance company has been quite nice.

There is a medical issue a day, can't make this stuff up, and Jackie sleeps again all day, restorative, restful, needed sleep. They are ratcheting down her narcotic painkillers, a prerequisite to making it back home. Jackie's happenings are moving in the right direction.

A Chance Meeting

From a chair, not a bed. Dust stirs outside the window. And then again. The small wisteria-like shoot that happened off the roof's edge goes crazy. One helicopter then another, the pad must be close. It's the helicopter to be in if need be. The kidney doc comes in, more blowing around, this time news that the kidneys really aren't back, that dialysis is. Nice try. Another line in another access, not a setback, just another medical mile in the recovery marathon, the one we were warned about, the one we can take.

Roll the orchestration down the hallway to the recessed elevator. Three people and Jackie board and then one more, Dr. Liam Ryan, the regular guy who for a living pops lungs in and out of people, sometimes more and then some, the transplant surgeon Jackie chanced meeting two months ago, chance meeting again. He looks around to the floral filter-valve masked young girl in the wheelchair, pauses, looks again, and says, "She looks good." Somehow hearing that from him means more than the rest of the people we chance meet traveling the corridors, not the passersby but the ones who pause and look, recognize and react, one of the many quiet celebrations going on in this dismal place where challenged bodies try to reclaim themselves.

Pass the inside fountain to the outside fountain where designated people meet. If only they could have been there to see Jackie see the sun. Such a simple thing, crossing that barrier between indoors and out but not so simple, the definition of success in Jackie's day. We find a shady spot, the castered pole and the lines, those life-giving tubes that follow her out. She pulls down the mask, closes her eyes, and lifts up her face. "Am I in the shade?" A chance meeting with the sun, with the outdoors. A chance meeting with life.

Dr. Clayton

From the day Jackie was born until the day she was grown and then some, one doctor knew her well, medically and otherwise. I like to say he raised her and wish I had captured all of his wisdom but we must have captured some. There's nothing that says, "Everything is going to be okay" like Dr. Clayton walking into a hospital room. He always said it's easier to do everything. Skill is in picking the right thing that works. And sometimes doing nothing. Discretion.

What saved Jackie's life was the ability of these high functioning people to exercise discretion at the highest level. Dr. Clayton came over from Pediatrics nearly every week, and sometimes every day to encourage Jackie. He told his colleagues, "Take good care of her, that's my friend in there."

Jackie's dad used to say that Dr. Clayton and Jackie's mother cheated the Grim Reaper and in a letter to thank this ICU for everything they have done for Jackie, I wrote, "Jackie's father says this hospital, her doctors, and her mother, and Jackie have for years cheated the Grim Reaper. This is what you are in this ICU, Cheaters of the Grim Reaper. You give people a chance to have a life out there. When you go home each and every day, you owe the world nothing more. You have given enough. We are witness. Thank you, though thank you feels too small. Still, I think you know." And Dr. Clayton must know.

Skin Barrier

The people in this place are constantly breaking the skin barrier. I'm thinking this entire hospital is about skin barriers, their natural obsession. Comes with the territory. You break yours, come on in. Or you come on in and they break it. Puncturing, slashing, tunneling… "What do you do for a living?" "I specialize in breaking the skin barrier." So today for Jackie, it was tunneling and tunneling hurts. Ouch.

They don't always put you to sleep for this stuff. Okay, they did numb the area and probably twilighted her but it wasn't pleasant. You know, that tugging you can feel and maybe throw in a little pain. Jackie's made friends with these folks in Interventional Radiology, she's been down for procedures so much. Today they did successfully tunnel that dialysis access into Jackie's chest wall guided by "imaging." Ouch again! Her dad calls it a "pig sticker." What's that? "A legendary dagger." He loves those terms. I try not to know about these things.

Unfortunately, tonight as her dad and I sit with her, it's about pain, the recalcitrant irritants to include neuropathic foot pain Jackie will kick in the butt through gaining strength, becoming more active, and in time, proper medication. If the place wasn't so clean, I would think we are hiking through mud, progress moves so slowly. But really not moving slowly. It's just the body, and they say Jackie's is progressing rapidly. Pippy, because of her pigtails to keep her hair away from the broken skin barriers, will soon be Jackie on her feet. She's getting skinny and her porcelain doll hands are coming back.

A Hospital Story

Hospitals create stories, good ones and bad ones, sensational ones, heart breaking, victorious ones. Here's a quick one. When Jackie was a preschooler, she and Jason, who was a teenager, met while hospitalized. They were both getting better from a cystic fibrosis flare-up, but were not ready to go home. Hospital stays were not so restricted back then and Jason would skateboard around and around the pediatric floor on his IV pole, one big circuit, waiting for discharge day. Skateboarding on IV poles was the hospital definition of fun. But then Jason got the office chair on casters from the nurse at the nurse's station and with Jackie in his lap, they made the circuit around and around the pediatric floor. "Wild times in Fairfax Hospital." That's what Jason said.

So many stories but not this week. Jackie's not feeling so great. The nurses say when patients are well and gone and return and walk in to visit, they don't recognize the patient. They recognize the family member walking in beside the patient and then they recognize the patient. Now that will be a story to tell once we get beyond the not feeling so great, and beyond.

Another Fuzzy Day

There's a fuzzy white filament on the computer screen, then a web of white, the cotton warmth covering Jackie. She's awake but she's down. Dr. Brown's scope travels in along the pink, moist corridors, open smooth tubules to those knobby remnants where her new lungs attach, one side and then the other, bilateral lung transplant, the complicated kind and now complications.

Watching the computer screen, listening and not understanding, words from a dainty lady with clear green eyes whom I would expect to spend time with a camera, never with a vacuum, but then add in airways, the unexpected doctor who also happens to be smart and sure and good at what she does, talking to the guy who's learning, the fellow from Paraguay. Welcome and thank you for helping our daughter.

Jackie's father watches from the door. His wheelchair can't compete with equipment and the coming together to figure this out, a collapsing lung lobe. I'm in here watching the stillness of Jackie and the movement of the scope. It's not red over here, but it is red over there, red-red, the color of you-know-what, the you-know-what they don't want to see in lung tissue. Then saline, the soft gentle slurp of cleaning out, opening things up down there, delicate things, the look of dainty again, airways this time. Not such bad news. Adjust the medications, take this one away, add that one in. This is transplant territory. Jackie's not asleep, just a light amount of sedation so as not to knock her out for the rest of the day. She's taking it like Jackie, accepting encouragement and the prompt to relax.

There've been enough procedures, enough sedation days already. Time to move forward, still, and again. Jackie looks at me, "This is too hard." It must feel good to say it like, "Why did I ever marry you?" or "I hate writing essays!" or "Life sucks!" when it really doesn't but saying it helps. "We will get through this together, Jackie. We get through everything together. We always work it out." It feels good to "go there" and today's the day to feel down. The bronchoscopy procedure is over. The minds kibitz and then turn off the complicated and make it simple and clear for us. Not so in every hospital. We know.

Everyone in this hospital explains well. It's what's set in place here. They've taken lessons on, good heavens, good communication. Jackie will be okay and Jackie will be bronched again next week. It's scary. It's not supposed to be this way. Oh, but it is. Gifts aren't free. We'll take them still. We'll take this gift of news today, not rejection but transplant tribulation. Jackie is back on the vent, an overnight rest. Thankful her face remains unencumbered by any contraptions such as breathing tubes though her trached neck still is. Thankful she'll be free of the ventilator soon, free of the hospital in just a few more tomorrows. Hope.

How do we unpaint someone from an ICU corner? We were trying to figure that out and dainty Dr. Brown was orchestrating it. Not to be fooled by the word "dainty," Dr. Brown is tough and competitive, competitive against death and that's some stiff competition. Jackie met her first in the emergency room two years back due to a cystic fibrosis lung exacerbation. Jackie remembers well that Dr. Brown did not flip the blinding examination lights on but sat beside Jackie in a bind in the dark and began to get to know her.

A doctor-patient relationship extraordinaire developed over the months and when the disease of cystic fibrosis turned so terribly mean and tried to take Jackie from us, Dr. Brown was there to say, not quite. She took care of Jackie at that point and would take care of Jackie again and again and we knew it. I was thankful to be the mom. It somehow felt like they were carrying the heavy burden and were prepared for it.

Jackie had good days sitting up in a chair, two not three people helping her move along from the bed. She remained on the ventilator by way of tracheostomy for that added breathing support until that one lung lobe settled down, which did not get us down. Still, neuropathic pain plagued her and we collectively prayed it would settle down and Jackie could truly move beyond suffering. This was not Jackie's first time though surely the worst time and I thought of a hospital story from age twelve.

Days Inn

Every mom needs a Days Inn. When Jackie was twelve, she had a dramatic intestinal surgery at Johns Hopkins University Hospital. Her surgeon showed up later in People Magazine as being one of the ten most important people in Ronald Reagan's life. He had been the daily hospital rounds doctor hand-picked for Nancy Reagan when her husband was shot. Two weeks after the surgery and Jackie was so far from recovering I was losing it. At that hospital at that time, they medicated the pain to the maximum, into the Twilight Zone, and got the patient up and walking.

Around ten p.m., a nurse pierced the heaviness, I needed a break, I had to get out of there for a night, to take a cab at the front door to the Days Inn Harbor Place. I went down to the entry to the line-up of cabs and got in one. Right away we came upon an old guy urinating on the street. And then, knowing the exact steady route from the harbor at the edge of Baltimore to Johns Hopkins Hospital, I knew. The cab guy ran me all over town. Baltimore. I sat frozen. Then he made his way to the Days Inn Harbor Place, "I don't take no hospital vouchers." I emptied my pockets into his hand and scooted out.

As I entered the hotel, I caught sight of the bar down the right corridor, so I headed there first with my small suitcase, project bag, and purse and plopped them down by the bar stool. A glass of wine and by the second, it was on them as they found out why I was there. The guy to my left was a businessman from Scranton, Pennsylvania and we bantered back and forth about raising his family in Scranton, of all places. My only experience there was stopping for gas, a fill up by a guy with a prison release ankle monitor on. All in fun, he defended Scranton. I asked for fried mushrooms but the kitchen was closed and all of a sudden even still, a huge basket of fried mushrooms appeared in front of me. Wow, the Days Inn. Not the hospital.

I suddenly caught sight to the right a weathered lady slipping onto the stool, a scraggly grey straw-haired toothless odorous homeless lady asking me if she could have some of the mushrooms. Of course, gladly. She ate them alone, gladly. She and I began to talk and the Scranton businessman left. I looked up and found the lights had slipped off and everyone had slipped out unnoticed, just the two of us into the night in the dimness.

She was going to kill herself that night, jump off a high place and I was going to talk her out of it. Where should she begin to save herself as I persuaded her? I suggested finding a dental school in Baltimore and getting a free remake of her teeth. She explained that her sister had a perfect life with her family in North Carolina, married to a doctor. She told me she had been an artist so I told her that her sister's life was way too predictable and boring and her life was much more interesting. Really? She did make an attempt at believing it.

She was so down and I tried to think of anything to give her hope and finally she said, easy for me, Bo Derek that I was. Now I may have been a lot of things but I was no Bo Derek, a hot bathing suit model from the 1980s. Even so, this homeless lady and I connected. I suppose in a way, I too was homeless that night.

Hours later, the businessman approached from a distance down the corridor and motioned me over. I picked up my bags and went. He said he could not sleep because he knew what I was doing, I could not save her. He grabbed my bags and led me away to the front desk. My credit card did not work so he wanted to pay for my hotel room, I knew with the right intentions.

We sorted it out on the phone with my husband, no cell phones back then, and he was determined that they give me a room near the front desk. This gentleman grabbed the key and led me down, unlocked the door and dropped my three bags by the window, went back to the door and commanded that I not go back down that corridor, he needed to be able to sleep that night.

I settled in and called my husband. What the heck was going on? It crossed my mind, a not-so-funny episode of Cheers, that bar sitcom also from the '80s. That short sleep that night felt long in the quiet of the Days Inn. I thought when I opened the room door in the morning, a slump of homeless woman would lay across the threshold and fall in at my feet. I opened carefully and tiptoed out, bags in hand, and took a cab, this time directly back to the hospital. Every mom needs a Days Inn.

Three weeks in and Jackie was much improved, I took a cab away again to grab a bite of Baltimore delight. When I got into the cab, broad daylight to be sure, the driver asked immediately about the hospital stay. He started in and not quietly, a preacher posing as a cab driver. "She need to be home! She need to be on that phone with her friends! She need to be going to school! She need to be well! Do you mind if my church pray for her?" Baltimore, a city surely full of personality. He was right. Get us home! Get our girl back to her life! And we did.

I continued to scribble on paper towels in Jackie's CardioVascular ICU room, thoughts and ideas echoing in my mind, captured in the moment or lost forever in split seconds. Composing at home each night somehow contributed to my ability to sleep and be present for Jackie the next day. This day, her dad wrote.

Compensation, a writing from Jackie's dad

Wow, what a summer. Thankfully, it is almost over and fall will soon begin. My father died in mid-September when I was a young child. I have always loved the spring for the obvious reasons of better weather and the proverbial rebirth of life but my dislike for fall had to do with the negative emotions connected to my father's death. But now there will be joy in the fall when my bonnie lass returns to the warm embrace of her home. The falling leaves and the cool air will no longer be companions of death but of life. Mr. Emerson has an essay on compensation, which seems to be appropriate.

We may not always be given what we want or need at a specific point in our lives but life, at least it seems so to me, has a way of compensating us in other ways. I have been compensated twice now in the fall, the first time when Jackie survived her birth trauma and now having survived her lung transplant. Isn't life amazing?

I look forward to the crisp air and the falling leaves; they will be auguries of life, of the new life my daughter will be embarking upon with renewed energy and vigor. What a testament to her spirit. Twice now, I have been witness to her indomitable will to live. I am so proud of this amazing human being for her zest for life, for the many friends she has, and for her desire to be a productive member of our society in spite of the hand life dealt. What a gift I was given to be her father. I truly have been compensated.

Jackie's brother landed back in town a third time, being able to take brief stints from his doctoral work even with the school year launching. They, like everyone else, were understanding and thoughtful. His field of study involves math and the brain very much like what Jackie was going through, all about the numbers and a bit more. He also wrote.

A Distraction

My mom wanted me to share a new "technology" that has emerged in the past few years. As I sat with Jackie, I tried to ease her discomfort, from aches and itches and pains, by entertaining her not with ideas that she enjoys, but ones that I enjoy. I figured her lack of interest would balance my over-exuberance to make a fine tale. Thus, we spoke of CRISPR. If you haven't heard of it, do some Googling because it's awesome.

CRISPR, often called CRISPR/Cas9 (/crisper kas 9/), is a DNA editing technology. It's basically an enzyme. It comes from certain types of bacteria, forming a crucial part of the bacterial immune system. Just as we protect ourselves from microbial mischief, bacteria fight off viruses. Viruses are little protein-coated packets of DNA, or DNA's cousin RNA.

What CRISPR does is recognize viruses. A lot like

one magnet attracts another, it finds and attaches to specific sequences of DNA (e.g. ATCCGTCAAG), which it knows from previous experience to belong to a malicious virus. Then, its partner in crime-fighting, Cas9, chops up the DNA and renders the virus unable to replicate.

Geneticists are super smart and they realized they might be able to take advantage of this powerful DNA-target-and-destroy bacterial immune system. So, they've started experimenting with CRISPR/Cas9 as a potential way to perform gene therapy. In brief, the molecules would enter human cells, target specific sequences of DNA, and change those sequences in certain ways. The ultimate goal is a cure, a genuine cure, for all hereditary disease.

From Huntington's disease to cystic fibrosis and muscular dystrophy, experiments are being performed at this moment on mice and rats and monkeys and even humans with promising results thus far. We may not see a cure in our lifetimes, but something similar to CRISPR/Cas9 will likely be responsible for a dramatic change in the fortune for a great many people. Isn't that awesome?

Having gone to Vanderbilt University with the mostest, Byron had become a minimalist with the leastest. He enjoys riding his bike to Boston University, studying long hours, working in a laboratory with equipment like this oversized multi-capable microscope resting on a pressurized air table to compensate for vibrations such as from traffic out on the road below. His work is a story in itself. The following was his favorite story of all that I wrote.

The Unlikely

I will never forget the night Jackie became so sick. I will never forget the day I looked at my daughter and knew, her look was going to change. Every day, her look slipping away, the changes of illness. Who else sees that? Who sees, and perhaps without distraction, a patient in a bed, the same bed, every day? Not the doctors, they do rotations. Not the nurses, they do "three 12's."   Not anyone but who? The mother and the unlikely.

A few years ago at discharge, Jackie completed a questionnaire. "Who had the most impact on your stay?" Jackie picked the unlikely. This person smiled an animated smile every day, in fact three times a day. We were sitting in that room and realizing the truth, his work wasn't so much about food though he brought food. He brought unencumbered kindness and encouragement three times a day, every day like no one else in that hospital. And the pressure these people must be under not to deliver food with an accidental touch of food poisoning. Imagine. Well, don't imagine.

This stay, and it's just a stay, Jackie has not eaten for weeks, not meals three times a day, but the food service lady, she notices, she watches, she waits like the mother, every day. Then all of a sudden meals, scrawny ones, pureed ones, chopped ones. They come. Untouched, they go. Then one day, "That's my baby girl in there, glad to finally see her eating."   I look up, startled, the only person along with me in this whole hospital who sees Jackie every day, off on weekends but weekends don't count if you've ever been in a hospital.

She "gowns up" and comes in to put that tray down, removing herself from that remote hallway to meet the sick girl she's watched get back that well look. There's something between us. She and I know, we were there, both of us, just us every single day. "I'm coming to your house when she gets out of here because I have to see her, she's my girl." Today Jackie bumped me out of the comfortable sleeper chair and such a simple thing, she ate a meal, part of a meal, with enjoyment, one of the many things that disappear in an ICU, or dwindle away... for a stay that is.

And then Jackie wrote.

Jackie here

I don't have as good of a way with words as my mom or dad but I'll try my best. My brother, Byron, is in town so the whole family is hanging out tonight. It's been a while since all four of us have been together. It's been almost three months since my hospitalization in June.

It's a weird feeling but every morning I wake up and hope for night again because that means another day has passed and I'm closer to going home. I want to be home so badly, in the comfort of my own house, in my own room, in my own bed. I want to go out to dinner with my friends again, walk again, work again (yea, I miss work!), live again. I know it will happen. My dad recently sent me a text that really helped me on a day I kept asking, "Why me?" Here's a little bit of it:

"You have a whole different perspective on life. CF has probably caused you to pull every last bit of living out of your life. That is why your friends love you. You grab the gusto. In a way you were given a gift of life. I think many people go through life half asleep, they just exist from day to day. You have had a lot of fun. I have seen it and paid for some of it. When you value life, as I know you do, you keep going to preserve your life. No matter the odds, you keep moving forward and you don't give up trying." So I keep fighting and will never stop until the last breath leaves my body.

Twice

We raised Jackie
We kept her safe
We organized and managed her life
We advocated, we disciplined and consequenced her
We helped her develop her skills and taught her to use her mind
We enjoyed her childhood

Then Jackie grew up
She kept herself safe
She organized and managed her own life
She advocated, she disciplined and rewarded herself
She utilized her skills and controlled her own mind
Jackie lived her life

Then yank, hurl, sheer and suddenly
The medical world kept Jackie safe
They organized and managed her life
They advocated, through discipline they stabilized
her
They utilized their skills and saved her
Jackie lived because of them

Now Jackie is recovering
She is helping keep herself safe
They with Jackie are organizing and managing her
life
She is advocating, and disciplining her own recovery
She will utilize her skills to determine her future
Jackie is living her life again

An Old Snare

~~~~~~~

When Jackie started high school, she used to sneak
out of her window until her brother taught her to
sneak out of her dad's home office door. The side window screen from her bedroom had hit the ground
too many times. One night, she called my cell phone
from her cell phone and I asked why she was calling
me from her bedroom. Pause. She passed her phone
to the police officer and I flung myself out of bed. She
and her friends and "an older boy" were at a park by
their high school swinging on swings, trespassing.

When the police approached, they did not run. They were not drinking alcohol or causing trouble, just swinging.

When I got there to retrieve Jackie, I recognized the officer from having worked in the alternative school in the courthouse. We talked about the eighteen-year-old, the last one standing there, the one who wasn't just getting a trespassing warning. I said, "He could have run. He didn't." The officer let him go and every time Jackie saw him at a party, this new adult told Jackie to thank her mom for getting him out of that snare. Moms deal in snares and thankful myself to have helped Jackie get out of her snares, medical and not medical.

Heidi Dalton

Heidi Dalton who got Jackie out of the snare with ECMO is in the ICU again, back from Arizona engaging in her monthly consulting at Fairfax Hospital's Heart and Vascular Institute and planning to visit with Jackie, to take a picture to include in an article and share at a conference in a presentation. Jackie needs that picture, too, the successful next to the successful.

Though she will always be the ECMO expert Dr. Heidi Dalton, we often, evermore, and affectionately refer to her like a smushed together first name, "HeidiDalton." ECMO, Extra Corporeal Membrane Oxygenation, may sound fun but it isn't. What a contrast to the last time we saw her, the day Jackie was attached to those external lungs, key to her survival.

This time, Jackie is up.

Heidi Dalton told Jackie's dad she developed an interest during her early days in medicine by making extra money spending nights sitting with patients who were assisted by heart/lung machines. She spent the better part of her career at hospitals in Washington, DC and then moved to Arizona and began consulting. What a twist for her to spin off on her own and wind back to our area with Innovative ECMO, our good fortune.

Christopher King is ECMO-accomplished himself. People say Dr. King has that rare and right intelligence to save lives. Amazing Dr. King met amazing Jackie. He is gracious and unassuming, seems shy, and he is smart. He explained this complex transplant and recovery process understandably but when he wrote about what happened in his industry's journal, we understood that we didn't quite understand, and didn't need to. Dr. King has authored numerous publications, lectured at national conferences, and serves on the American College of Chest Physicians. Am I bragging? Yes.

The day came when Jackie's physical therapist, Jonathan, left. He had an itch to move to outpatient services. He's around Jackie's age and encouraging and funny. He said if she saw anyone wearing mismatched scrubs, "Code B" for brown as in a poopie accident happened, an accident someone had on him the third day of work there. Jonathan helped Jackie surprise herself, to move more than the day before. With their good-byes, Jonathan told Jackie, "You're my favorite patient and in my whole career, I think you always will be."

Into the Hallway

Before Jackie launched out into the hallway, another patient already had, circling around and around followed by the ventilator cart and physical therapist. Jackie dreamed tearfully of being where this young lady was and told her doctor so. Simply stated by Dr. Brown, "She has her own journey." Soon, the mother of Anya came to Jackie's door with a note in hand, the website of Anya's journey.

Anya is older than Jackie by nearly two decades and she has had two lung transplants. She is not well. Rejection is challenging her. Anya's mother began visiting Jackie, bringing her gifts and offering encouragement. Anya from afar and her mother from close have inspired Jackie to make it out of that bed and into the hallway, to make it out of that hospital and into her life.

Jackie is doing her best. It is not about relearning. It is about reclaiming, moving away from "profoundly weak," the deflating term we no longer hear. It is about getting out of that room so we, too, begin circling, seeing what is going on out there, Jackie in the wheelchair, the therapists, mom and IV pole. "Code Walk" is not much of a risk for the old and crinkly on this unit but an alert call when a patient escapes. Jackie and I contemplate "Code Wheel" except the back stairwell won't accommodate us, though the sight of the outdoors through the plate glass window at the end of the hallway tempts us to try.

Jackie and I have so many funny stories. I once drove into the hospital grounds to find a stooped old guy, IV pole-turned-cane in one hand, ciggie in the other, gown and exposed back side flapping in the wind, walking away down the sidewalk. I, too, kept moving along, sympathetically. Then another story not from this fine place, we had been in a few, where a guy disappeared from his room. Police found him down the road at the local karaoke bar. He got out of that relatively quiet place and we will, too, one day soon.

Quiet

~~~~~~~~

Quiet, that wicked concoction that ignited our daughter's lungs and sought to throw her into unrecoverable medical madness. The quiet now, the quiet of beating that madness, the quiet of recovery. Back in Jackie's room, still random sleeplessness, itches and ouches, muted taste buds, a little fever here, blood tinged cough there, still no real voice, all part of the slow climb back, these four walls and quiet.

The mom, the fixer of everything with words, also quiet. Jackie uses a few choice words at me. It gets a little crazy in there, everyone on this mission including the lovely-dispositioned and appreciated nurse in here this day, her hijab giving a clue she does not cuss, excuse me for saying but I don't think she does. She laughs a small uncomfortable laugh, sympathetic and kind.

When I get home, I tell Jackie's father and he texts her, "If a girl cusses and she has no voice, is it still cussing?" Leave it to her dad. I have to remember Jackie owns this. She borrowed me for a time but she is almost twenty-five and getting her life back and I am ready to give it back to her. "Quiet," a book I love, about introversion. Not something to fix, who you are. I used to think I could honor the introvert in me screaming to come out but then I'd forget. Maybe I could be an introvert the next day. In that room in those hours, a real opportunity to practice introversion, silence that says so much, the introvert who needs to stop and think and not speak, to allow Jackie to rest and recover and not get upset.

When I got upset, I clung to the respiratory therapists. They were beautiful, male or female, angels day or night coming in to work the machines to work the numbers, to get them just right, to get the lungs just right. They were patient with patients and progress, numbers and machines. I used to say as a teacher, I worked with my students every day and over time, knew them well.

The respiratory therapists work with lungs every day and know them well and those respiratory therapists I clung to knew Jackie's lungs well. Craig suffered lunch interruptions if I saw him in the cafe as I sought the hope he as an insider could give. He remained calm and encouraging through my internal emotional earthquakes and for that I am grateful.

CHAPTER SIX

SEPTEMBER MEANT
ONE HUNDRED DAYS

After nearly one hundred days and into September, Jackie got moved down the hallway and around the corner. Dr. Williams, in critical care demand in other areas of the hospital, made his way to the CVICU to see for himself how Jackie was progressing, and offered a few fresh ideas like moving Jackie to another room, one filled with sunrises and sunsets as she got better.

The nurse night fairies made the transformation in the wee hours. It was time to say good-bye to the operating room across the way, literally and figuratively. We moved next to that plate glass window and the stairwell escape route and glanced at each other tempted to bolt, bored over a quiet weekend. We proposed rather a walker race-down-the-hallway challenge since the ninety-year-old guys had more walker experience and Jackie was new at it but young, thus leveling the playing field.

We preferred the more secure feeling of the bustle of

weekdays. Weekends, we noticed the parking garage down below lay half empty as people reassembled their lives out there in preparation for the coming week. Maybe Jackie could get outside again, too, and enjoy the weather of the final days of summer. She broke the boredom in the meantime by ordering clothes online in anticipation of her upcoming rehabilitation, another hospital and more strangers.

Strangers

There's this whole stranger component to life. There's just a whole lot more people in this world beyond the outer circle and few in the inner circle. It's logistical. What amount of our lives is spent with strangers? Maybe we unknowingly select jobs based in part on this, the lawyer who meets and greets and gets to know for a time, the store clerk who meets and greets and that's it, the teacher who has parents and guests entering and exiting their rooms.

We're all used to intermingling with faces we don't recognize, those whom the brain does not yet compute. Medical conditions create forced entries into stranger encounters and often a steady stream of them. Not only do these strangers learn about our private selves, they learn about our private physical selves in short order and it's disconcerting. What's the definition of a disease? Moving, often suddenly, into a stranger world of being told what to do with time and body, being bossed around. Really?

What's hard for me is crossing that threshold into a new medical arena, standing at that entryway, looking up, taking a deep breath, and entering. Wish it wasn't so... but it is so, no fighting it. Lean into it. Whether self or child or brother or mother or friend, just step and then step again and enter.

And then we found ourselves in this position in life... frozen, listening, relying and Jackie, or rather her body, somehow cooperating and now all of us together adapting, appreciating, the reliance on strangers. At what point are they no longer strangers? Certainly not her beloved doctors, respiratory therapists, familiar caregivers. But the ticket lady at the garage exit nodding each time, maybe no longer a stranger. The ophthalmologist who worked all day and came to Jackie's room at ten o'clock at night, twice, because he was on call and her eyes were in a delicate state, a possible eye infection, this stranger entering the room with his metal suitcase full of ophthalmology tools assessing, the stranger who won't need to come back. Others enter, their own respective specialty, respecting these people whose paths we will not again cross.

For Jackie now finding her stride, a big part of each evening, learning who her night nurse will be. New caregivers mean new communications about what works and what doesn't work in settling her in, seeking healing rest at the hands of strangers. She's good at it by now, such large amounts of time with the unfamiliar performing what is for her familiar.

The powerhouse nurses whose central nervous systems take on patients on the edge, are not often in Jackie's room anymore. A pool of nurses whose central nervous systems may not accommodate the frenzy, yet nurturing and thorough and thoughtful, making getting well happen. Now more often, new to Jackie, strangers. Sickness means needing them. Recovery means minding needing them and we look forward to the time when Jackie is ready to come home no longer in the care of strangers.

Jackie remained in the CVICU, the CardioVascular Intensive Care Unit, the high nurse-to-patient ratio meeting the demands of her care. Though she continued to see Dr. King, the transplant pulmonologist, she did not continue to see Dr. King, the intensivist. He as ICU intensivist would stop in anyhow just to speak words of encouragement to this precious success story but maybe not on days that were abuzz. The CVICU, where the sickest patients undergo the top medical care such as the most difficult lung transplants, sometime perform six in one week with sometimes a dozen transplant patients in there at one time. Dr. King would be a little busy. And so would the other transplant intensivist pulmonologists on their team. Fortunately for all of us, there are smart people out there. Dr. Brown would remain evermore the constant in Jackie's transplant care, nevermore a stranger.

Birthday Week

Jackie's birthday is this week, September 16th and the best gift, making it out of the other ICU room and the prospects of making it out of this ICU room in the back corner, making it out of this CVICU altogether. Jackie can see and she mentions, so many patients so lifeless. The stillness in their beds purposeful, maybe medication-induced comas or maybe restorative

sleep, the givers of care and receivers of care, the ra-
zor-focus meeting the demands, heart and lung and
this week, a lot of lung they tell us. This is a serious
place where split seconds and split decisions meet
and sometimes collide, as I can tell walking down the
hallway. My eyes attempt to look straight ahead but I
get it, pull back tears, the so very sick.

Protocols are carefully followed out of need and out
of respect. Strangely, following them makes me feel
welcome and comfortable as a visitor, like I somehow
belong here doing my part in this respiratory sensitive place, careful not to bring in flowers or cell phone
noise. As the Director of Nursing, Mickey reminds
me this is also a place for celebration. Jackie smiles
when he stops in daily in celebration. He wants her
to celebrate her birthday here, the happy place, the
place where Jackie reclaimed her ability to be happy
and to celebrate.

She will be twenty-five and the Director of Nursing
will be a brave soul. He'll allow, gowned and gloved,
twenty-five impressive and responsible young adults,
friends of Jackie's, to throw her a CVICU room party. Jackie has ordered cupcakes from Cupcaked from
smart Kristina in our smart little town of Clifton.
The sign in her store: "She believed she could so she
did." The crowd in Jackie's room will decorate and
celebrate, eat and pile high for an all-encompassing
birthday photo. The window from the outside, bal-
loons in reverse, "Happy Birthday!"

We were so easily reminded of where we were as autumn
crept in. As Jackie reclaimed herself, intermittent unrest

and discomfort followed intermittent rest and comfort followed intermittent unrest and discomfort. Rest and comfort would win but not yet.

Easy Street

There lives a title in my head, "Looking for Easy Street." Maybe there is no Easy Street to write about but wouldn't it be nice? Jackie is feeling anxious tonight, part of weaning off the ventilator. Thank goodness when our breathing is challenged, we instinctually feel anxious, like that coming-upon-the-bear-in-the-forest-fear response. Let's hope so. Jackie and I have been texting tonight to bring comfort. Wish I could be there but hospitals separate people like Jackie and me tonight and they certainly are scenes for anxiety.

When Jackie was born, I couldn't escape feeling anxious myself and called our minister stumbling over why I was calling and he said, "You will experience God in a way you don't even know exists right now," a flutter of hope in the midst of despair. In the depths of that time, I wrote, "It is strange to be lying in bed and all of life is darkness and beyond grasp and that one small glimmer says, 'God is here.' The suffering that life offers instills in us this silence." And now I think, sometimes silence is all that's left. I find comfort in silence and I want Jackie to, as well. Her birthday party is over and friends will continue to come but I pray she will feel the sense of calm I've seen in her going through this over these months. And pray breathing will bring her not anxiety but comfort, a little piece of Easy Street.

What Jackie Can Do

~~~~~~~~

Jackie can almost use her voice.
She can walk a short distance with help.
She can sit up on the side of the bed.
And pivot with help to a chair.
She can cross her legs.
And move her arms about.
Brush her teeth and comb her hair.
She's eating partial meals.
Jackie can breathe on her own during the day.
To leave the ICU, she has to be able to breathe
on her own during the night
And surely before the month's end.
She's fragile and has to be careful for now.
But it will all come back.
She continues to boss her mom around.
And enjoy her dad's sense of humor.
We are lucky ones.

We were counting on this anxiety being the last vestige of this traumatic event, the body firing back up, purging toxins, making plans. We knew she was surrounded by people who could help. I was reminded of our pulmonologist Dr. John Osborn, who with Dr. Clayton saw Jackie through childhood. We relied on both of them as one or the other did have to go home for dinner sometimes and did need a turn at taking vacations much as we did not want them to.

I spoke with Dr. Osborn throughout. We met Dr. Osborn when Jackie was little and in a medical bind. Her dad and I were in a quandary until we heard that assuring voice on the other end on that 1 a.m. phone call. Jackie led her life with interruptions rather than living an interrupted life because of Dr. Osborn. He was aggressive but not rough. His news was never bad news because we knew he knew, and we listened.

Dr. Osborn made having this disease not hard. He reached in and he reached out. We went through medical highs and lows, tenacious street fighters beating cystic fibrosis. Though he moved miles away, the miles did not prevent Dr. Osborn from answering his phone once again, reminding us, as always, to press forward.

Jackie's coworkers, from her new-to-the-United States German company Lidl, came to visit her in the ICU, again. Lidl, in the news, was beginning to open their stores here, having been in Europe for over forty years. "With 10,000 stores in 27 countries, designed to deliver high quality at low prices and an efficient shopping experience." Is this an advertisement for them? Yes, this is so. Their signage: "Welcome to Lidl. We want you to be a part of it." They wanted Jackie to be a part of Lidl and for that, we were thankful.

My nightly updates developed competition with Jackie's photo-share postings so I appealed for her to contribute to our update group.

Jackie: My Nurses

It's Jackie again. I made it out to the Healing Garden. A few nurses came along and they loved an excuse to get outside! It was a beautiful day. Mickey, he's in charge of the CVICU, came and a great guy! He's the one who allowed my birthday party! I will definitely miss the nurses when I get out of here. They were and still are an integral part of my recovery and help keep me motivated. Ones I don't have that day pop in to say hi, they tell me how great I'm doing, they clapped when I walked for the first time, they make me comfortable, they make me feel safe.

If you ever doubted what a nurse does, come spend a day here in the CVICU and you'll have a whole new perspective. My friend is an ICU nurse and I would always ask her if she was bored having only one patient at a time. She laughed and said there were always things the patient needed. I became that patient and realize there is no down time as an ICU nurse, or any nurse for that matter. So thank you to all the nurses out there and my nurse friends, Jen, Sam, Molly, Caitlyn, thank you.

Jackie spent nights off the ventilator with the tracheostomy still in place. We spent evenings with her and my nightly writing fell by then onto paper like melted butter.

Cell Phones

~~~~~~~~

I'll make a simple observation tonight and that is about cell phones. Cell phones create this three-way call convenience dynamic. Our friends this week shared how the dad needs to reach the mom and gets the daughter to call the mom because the mom is more likely to pick up if the daughter calls even though the dad, not the daughter, wants to talk to the mom.

We'll call Jackie's brother and he won't answer so we get Jackie to call because he will answer if she calls even though we're trying to reach him. I was sitting on the front porch at home this week and daddy Byron from in the house called my cell phone and I didn't answer so then Jackie sent me a text. I got off my call and saw that Jackie from the hospital texted me, "Where are you? Dad needs you." Dad in the house is getting Jackie in the hospital to get me off the front porch?

Jackie once, in her hospital room, needed help and texted that her nurse must be caught up in another room and could I call the nurses' station, a voice for her to get someone to come to her room. From our house, I got a nurse in Jackie's unit to go to Jackie's hospital room.

We think next week Jackie will get her voice back and won't need to text me to reach someone at the nurses' station but thank heavens in the meantime we all have cell phones. Could we live without cell phones and this three-way call convenience?

One night when we were visiting with Jackie, she and her dad and aunt were engaged in some sort of banter. I had not scribbled any thoughts that day so I pulled myself away along with the bedside table on wheels-turned-writing-surface and this dropped off my fingers.

Love

I love being Jackie's mom. Love, yes, and it feels good to say it this way, the public side of "I love you." I think about how Jackie's life was saved, almost have to make myself remember all that took place here to get us to this point tonight, a sleepover in room 212, just for fun. Every so often a conversation between us, I remember how a drug caused exaggerated facial tics and they got her off immediately never to use again, or how they had to open up Jackie's chest twice in a row, a below-the-breast vast clam shell incision like a "w", no ribs broken but "creak" I imagine as they lifted, the first time to transplant and then again to get things cleaned up in there. Twice? she questioned. True indeed.

Her dad and I want to read the hospital notes sometime, hundreds of pages though just the procedure part to sort out the convoluted blur. No jumping too far ahead of ourselves. Jackie's dealing with nausea the past couple of days like right after the Healing Garden visit outdoors, losing her meal into the blanket-turned-catching-bowl cupped in my hands.

There's something every day, can't make this stuff up, but it passes. Battle wounds are still healing; the focus: putting that ventilator to rest completely. She'll keep this nifty trach throat device for a while, a safety measure that beats needing to be intubated again or even beats getting another trach, can't just pop those things in and out one after another. The docs are being cautious. They carry the decisions and worries. I'm here to enjoy Jackie, bring fun food from home and comfortable clothes she's now wearing, and to laugh at the family banter.

Jackie handles her care with her doctors herself now. They must have a bond, such a victorious exertion to save Jackie, our gift to them. Please take her, take her completely, do what you must to save her. Jackie reminds me on occasion, "Mom, this is not happening to you."

I tell her story through my story and though this disease is not happening to me, being her mom, it's raw. I've always liked the Patricia Yearwood song, "I would've loved you anyway. I'd do it all the same. Not a second I would change. Not a touch that I would trade. Had I known my heart would break..." except guess what? My heart didn't break. And I love being Jackie's mom.

Jackie survived more bouts of nausea. I often thought to myself, "Not the day that we want but the day that we have. Please let the day go by." I also thought about the high level of constant problem-solving going on and my favorite message to my students back in the day. "Just because it's hard doesn't mean you don't do it." Doing what's hard expands us and doing what's hard medically expands all of us, I reminded myself.

Nothing worked one weekend to counter the nausea and with the backdrop a new lung transplant, the body teetering towards recovery, they had to counter it. Maybe it was a stomach virus that would go away and leave her alone and I called in the night in hopes that it had. The two pretty people, Jackie and Dr. Brown, conferred that Monday morning and rearranged the anti-rejection and anti-nausea drugs and Jackie pulled out of it. Dr. Brown remained in high gear orchestrating Jackie's transplant recovery.

I attended a "town hall" dinner in the hospital that night. At first, too many personnel and too few patrons were in attendance until I realized once the administrator began to speak, I had by accident crashed a medical staff event. I finished eating and tried to slip out only to pass by the Senior Director of Building & Support Services, Earnest. He was one of the "Mom in the Hallway" lucky ones I had approached about his role there, in charge of everything not medical, the physical plant. He wrangled me into speaking before the group before I left.

I extemporaneously summarized Jackie's journey over the years with this hospital, how we witnessed it grow into a well-oiled machine. We lived it and we knew and they needed to hear it from us. While speaking, I kept my eyes on Carolyn, a thoracic surgery nurse practitioner who met Jackie at the worst, and smiled the whole time knowing of her progress. She had written in Jackie's journal that patients like Jackie give them a chance to stretch themselves and to believe. She wrote that Jackie had grit. Those past days of nausea demonstrated that Jackie had grit and that Jackie also believed. Her father wrote.

Convergence, another writing from Jackie's dad

~~~~~~~

Convergence is just a way to say there are long series of events in our lives that lead to good or bad outcomes, some of that series out of our ability to control and the only thing to control is how we handle what life sends our way, to be cognizant of what is in our power to control and accept what is beyond our power to control.

We handle our trials and tribulations based on experiences in our past and then we have these events that converge to cause problems. We handle the problems that life throws at us based on our perception of what the events are and how they impact us. We may think of a horrible event as beyond our ability to cope but we really don't yet have the perspective to truly understand if this was a life shattering event or a life-shaping event. We should not allow life to shatter us but look at each experience as a convergence of events that form our understanding about life and ourselves.

Into September, though still in the CVICU, Jackie began to have better days. Nausea was better and her bronchoscopy brought good news. I had always said that I was doing as well as Jackie looked and she was looking well. On a best day, she blocked the valve on her trach and with her voice, glory be, spoke on the phone about a small investment she needed to move. She planned her post-discharge pulmonary rehabilitation (weight training with a twist), and talked about bedroom renovations to come home to.

Jackie: Looking Forward To...
a double size bed
wearing street clothes
taking a tub bath
driving my car

spending money at a store
going to friends' apartments
mom's cooking
shoes fitting
my own four walls
getting the trach out of my neck
getting taste buds back...

Jackie would be transferred to the rehabilitation hospital once she was off the ventilator for one week. Leaving the tracheostomy in place in case of emergency was not such great news, but the ventilator settings were turned off three-24's, closer and closer to being turned off seven-24's which would finally be the best news. She would also take with her the need for dialysis and hope remained for kidney recovery. Her father told her she could write on our update group that she couldn't wait to cuddle fuzzy kittens and puppy dogs, that she loved rainbows and butterflies and all of her friends and family would be just as happy. We had many small happy hospital stories and some bigger ones.

Ted

Ted's in pastoral care. He's been at the hospital for more than a decade so he's been coming to see Jackie more than a decade. He's seventy-some and kind and handsome, a gentleman. At first, Jackie would ask me to stay in the chair so pastoral visitors would be forced to stand and therefore not stay long.

Ted became important with time and faith-filled

visits, and she wanted him to know she was there and even wanted him to have a chair. Jackie's enjoyed the distraction of stories about his life and family through the years and she grew to appreciate the person, Ted. I always think of Ted as the marrying kind, fifty years too late.

East Coast to West

When Jackie was eight and visiting her Aunt Laura and Uncle Mark at Cherry Point Marine Air Station in North Carolina, she developed a high-grade intestinal obstruction, which can happen with cystic fibrosis and summer heat, sticky mucus and dehydration. The doctors on base medevac-ed her out to the hospital at the University of North Carolina Chapel Hill. Her uncle flew in the helicopter with her, her father and I drove down through the night around traps of road construction and heavy storming. The Raleigh/Durham Airport was put on delay to get Jackie through. Jackie lived there for five days, and her mother, too. Yes, we had been to Chapel Hill, North Carolina, but no, we had not. We scurried out of that town upon discharge.

Lots of grey matter, the specialist we met who backed Jackie out of this medical mess and set us on our way. When handed a new elementary class list that fall, I looked down at it and looked up at the principal who said, "I know what you went through this summer so I did you a favor." I'd had hard classes before, we all had, years when staring down at that new assignment, a slew of rough boys on that list.

One year, the little girl who had cancer and the little girl whose mother just died of cancer, I looked up at the principal, "I can't." He looked back, "You have to and you can." So I did.

Was I sorry that my teacher friends got those rough ones I didn't get that year? They were supportive and kind and didn't mind. We were up-close witnesses to each other's challenges, a coming together in a school of the incredible. How fortunate I spent ten years of Jackie's growing up years working there.

The year after that fresh summer memory, Jackie went back to that military base where she ran around so free and happy. Her Aunt Laura used to say Jackie could run the whole military base given a chance. They came up with a bright and simple idea, bake cookies to thank the medevac crew who had billed the event out as "a practice." Jackie and her aunt took the cookies over to find a room-filled meeting including the thank you guys. They stood up together, told the story, and Jackie and her aunt shared the cookies. The audience gave a standing ovation.

Very few people come back, very few people say thank you though they do surely think it. Back, not in a bind, just Jackie… and aunt, now Jackie's California connection. North Carolina memories on the military base were replaced by summer blasts living on the Outer Banks during those college years. Uncle Mark and Aunt Laura moved to California and thinking about going there makes being in the hospital a little less crazy! Making plans and planning on keeping them.

The Door Out

So many ICU's in this hospital, "Oh, that ICU is on the other side of the hospital." Really? This one is our ICU and we will be leaving it soon and it won't be ours anymore. Time to walk down new hallways where we can look left and right, pretend no more not to see what we can't help but see, near- tombed bodies and not such old ones lately. Awful.

Avoid ECMO lane, the side where alarms that know how to imitate panic are apt to sound. Can't help but notice the moving about down there, the life-saving ones who saved Jackie, saving again. Jackie, masked and ready, walker in front, wheelchair not far behind just in case, takes steps down the more quiet hallway. Maybe playing "Eye of the Tiger" as Jackie walks, that quiet echo of music somehow reaches those rooms, offering a sense that everything can become alright as it is for Jackie.

We pass Jackie's old room, someone else's turn to part from loved ones for a time. It was lonely back then, Jackie there but not there, unaware of the movement and hope in that operating room across the way. She keeps walking towards the door but not out the door yet. We round the corner heading back, steps increasingly more fluid and sure. The nurses comment, amazing, not thinking that they too are amazing. Let them enjoy the girl passing by, the girl they met weeks after they met her, caught first in that unimaginable life pause.

Sunshine spills into Jackie's room, empty spaces once taken by imposing machines, the ventilator, the last remnant of illness, gone. Time for us to go. Jackie is well. Her turn is over. She doesn't belong here anymore. The same applause we heard the day Jackie arrived in the ICU, someone in long illness, well and leaving, the notion that may one day be us and now it will be us, our ICU celebration.

We will have hospital bills as a reminder of what went on here. Chris from Blue Cross/Blue Shield, yet another angel, says he will manage them. There will be hand-holding, the rehabilitation hospital and case managers, transition specialists, people who will learn what happened to Jackie and will be a part of Jackie moving on to the life waiting out there for her, a life she is ready to get back to. She says she can feel it in her fingertips. Yes, amazing.

CHAPTER SEVEN

OCTOBER
JOURNEYED ALONG

By the first of October, we had journeyed together through so many medical miles, giving Jackie a chance in an isolating room not to be alone, living indeed with continued words of encouragement. Every day, I wanted to go as much as the day before, to gown and glove and live with Jackie within those four walls. Such an unreal existence but this existence was coming to an end as they planned to transport her by ambulance to rehab later in the week.

As I walked down the quiet corridors back to Jackie's room one Sunday afternoon, I said out loud to myself, "We're ready not to spend time in borrowed spaces." Hospital rooms are borrowed spaces, temporary homes by circumstance and we did our best to create out of Jackie's more than it was, a small living room for guests, a party room, a place to encourage Jackie onward towards home. We've climbed a long way out of this borrowed space and would one day in sight be in our own space, home and together again. We could see it. Grateful didn't begin to say it.

The liaison between the two places, hospital that transplants and hospital that rehabilitates, gowned and gloved and entered to allay fears, "It's going to be great!" We doubted it would be great. We didn't doubt it would be effective. Kidney dialysis and the trach collar would go with her. The night before this long anticipated day, in moving forward, Jackie looked back.

Jackie: Rehab Tomorrow

On June 13, my life forever changed. I was placed in a medically-induced coma with my mom and dad holding each one of my hands. I had one promise I wanted from the doctor and that was that I would wake up again. He promised me. Little did my family know, I would be listed for transplant 4 days later and in another 4 days a viable donor would be found. I was placed on ECMO, had numerous emergency surgeries on my abdomen and new lungs and my parents had to sign waiver after waiver, many of which said I only had a 50% chance of survival. But that's what I do, I fight and I survive. So here I am, 115 days later, on the eve of my discharge from the place I've called home all summer and into fall.

Off to rehab tomorrow to regain strength and independence. One step closer to home. None of the last 115 days would be possible without my donor and I will never forget that. I hope to meet my donor's family one day; I can write them a letter in June. I want them to know that I am living the best life I can with my new lungs and their son/daughter is living on through me and all the other lives they've saved. I am alive today because of their selflessness.

I also can't thank my friends and family enough. A major part of my recovery was knowing that I had so many people there supporting me. People I haven't talked to in years reached out to me. My friends came to visit me whenever they could, would just sit with me if I was too tired to talk, tell me about what I was missing out in the world, bring me food from the outside and even paint my toe nails [ahh!].

There is one other person who never failed to be by my side every single day and that is my mom. She did everything and anything I needed to heal and be comfortable. Without her, I wouldn't have made it through this sane. And I also can't forget my dad, of course. He continued to work hard for our family during all of this. I always looked forward to the days he came up; we have jokes and we just get each other. I pray my lungs continue to heal and thrive in their new body. And I pray my stubborn kidneys remember to work again soon.

The good-byes didn't feel real, but Jackie was ready. She slept the bumpity-bump gurneyed ride to Mount Vernon. The new space was impressive and the welcome seamless, yet at nightfall, I didn't want to leave Jackie and she didn't want me to leave her. What kind of sleep would it be, the newness of it all? Leaving the oddly comforting space, the CVICU, was a glide but settling into this new space felt like a heave. We could not find Jackie's cell phone charger, her cell phone being her lifeline to the familiar. With anticipation and trepidation, we forged on.

Snakes

We used to have a pet snake in a big aquarium on the floor and fed the pet snake mice from the pet shop. Once when I was buying a mouse for the snake (snakes have to eat, too), a guy was with the same store clerk buying a mouse for his tarantula and I asked him how he could have a tarantula. When a tarantula bites into a mouse, the interior of the mouse liquefies and I knew that. The guy asked me how I could have a snake. He was right. The pet shop mouse would meander in the snake cage for a quick minute and be eaten alive.

Once when construction was going on, a new house next door, field mice took cover in our house and we caught, barely, one running hard and fast down the hallway and fed it to the snake. That field mouse fought that snake hard and fast. The snake won but blood was shed. I looked in that snake cage and thought, I would rather be that mouse who has fought his way through life than the mouse that has lived comfortably in a pet store cage, then getting eaten alive. That field mouse was smart and "tried by life," making it in this world until given an unfair disadvantage in the snake cage.

I took our snake to a reptile pet shop, enough of snakes already, and when the shop-keeper reached in for the snake, it swallowed up the guy's thumb and he had to go to the back and immerse the snake in water for several minutes to get the snake to let go. I was proud of that snake.

Our snake cage aquarium remained empty at the

back porch door until that week when the three ducks we had would not allow us to catch them and put them in their cage. The kids and I were running around like ninnies trying to catch them before sunset and unsuccessfully and dad was laughing his you-know-what off. In the middle of the night, I awoke to a flurry of activity in the back yard and opened the bedroom door to find shadowy movements of fox on duck.

I ran down to the kitchen to find one lone duck on the final back step up. I grabbed a towel, opened the door, and lifted the willing duck into my arms. Apparently he did know where to find safe haven. I placed him, blood-tinged, into the empty aquarium cage and there he remained through the night after which I returned him, also, back to home territory, to the friend who had given us this bright idea of pet-keeping. Enough pets for us already, lesson learned.

Sometimes you have to fight and sometimes you have to find safe haven. Hospitals are where you do both. Jackie looks well. Her hair is thick and shiny and her skin is clear. Jackie is doing well. She's smart and ready, knows how to fight, knows when to find safe haven.

Forward Movement

Wow. We are here and moving forward. Rehab seems simple unlike intensive care, yet serious and important, too. There are lots of wide spaces in this place for people who can't walk but soon will. We don't want

Jackie here but it is the right place. She checks online, shoes for winter. "Jackie, your feet are still swollen. Better wait." She holds up one foot and then the other, "You may be right." She is reclaiming herself, figuring it out. It is up to her, the transplant diet like no sushi, her favorite, nothing raw, nothing potentially unwashed like lettuce, nothing outdated. Always seems to come down to food.

In spite of the food restrictions, the dialysis, the wounds, and whatever more, the real name of the game is the lungs and those lungs are good lungs. Someone took care of those lungs and it is Jackie's turn to take good care of them and she will. Hard to think about. Strange. Unexpected. Real. Appreciated. Thankful.

Jackie can walk short distances without the walker. She can transfer from a bed to a chair on her own. She grooms herself from a chair at the bathroom sink. And tires easily, having to pace herself. Her hands are shaky, a side effect of the medications but improving and will continue to. And she is finally fully weaning off the trach, minimal occasional breathing support, as she hoped. And though Mount Vernon Rehabilitation Hospital is pleasant, she is hoping to go home soon.

I stay with Jackie here all day and some nights, thankful for both the gurgling trach humidifier and the Brookstone Tranquil Sleep thunderstorm, the gift from dear Carmen. Dear Mo stays with Jackie's dear dad.

Mo

Mohamed came to the United States over ten years ago after being injured in the civil war in Sierra Leone, West Africa. He spent a year in recovery, one knee destroyed. Mo, healthy and well, walks with one leg straight. I felt bad when I asked him if he wanted us to rent bikes when we went to the beach but made up for it by renting a golf cart.

Mo says his slow recovery created empathy but I have a feeling Mo was born empathetic. Mo was born good. The rickety truck Mo was in, in the middle of a civil war his country was in, traveled all day to reach the hospital there. Mo's friend died along the way. They stopped the truck and dragged his friend's body into the woods and went on. "Why did they do that, Mo?" There were too many dead bodies at the hospital already.

Mo obtained asylum in the United States and is now an American citizen. Upon arrival here, he donated one of his kidneys to a relative and nearly died from an accidental cut into an artery. Mo grew up in the fields of West Africa, Daddy Byron grew up on the streets of Saint Louis, well not quite, but how strange their lives merged. Mo goes many places with us to help and to enjoy himself.

He went with us to Jackie's graduation at Radford University. During the ceremony, Mohamed stared across the rows of students and all about the grounds, complete disbelief that this could be real and affordable. We told him that one day his own children could attend a school like this. Mo has worked with us for nearly ten years and been married nearly half that long, his wife not allowed to come to America until recently.

Mo and his wife, Fatmata, describe medical care in their home country. Electricity access is rotated around the area as if in our area, "Springfield" today, "Vienna" tomorrow, "Chantilly" the next day. If medical care requires electricity, it doesn't happen during off-days.

People who can't afford medical care don't bother going to the hospital because if they do go, they are turned away. Mo has lived here always with friends and family to be a help and now he has a wife, long awaited hope for their own home and family. His wife and I hold conversations about the cost to replace a roof here, to refinish floors, or redecorate a room, unimaginable to her.

Mo has tripped over himself backwards, upside down, and every which way coming and going to help us during this tumultuous time. When Jackie comes home in one week, we won't need what the rehabilitation hospital suggests, finding someone to help. We have Mohamed. Mo is happy like Jackie is happy. They wake up that way.

A Ways Away

It feels a long way away, going to see Jackie, and a long way away, getting Jackie home. Mount Vernon, all the way to Route 1, too far to come, go, come, and go again. Her dad misses her. He wants her home. We are prepared. Who wouldn't be? In five days, it will be our turn. I almost stop by the Fairfax County Fire and Rescue Station to talk to them about how she is recovering, her lungs still fragile. Just thinking about being smart but then, they are smart enough so I keep driving and thinking.

This is life, imperfect, worth it. We will go on supporting Jackie as she breathes, walks and talks, smiles, and at times lowers her head, finger to eye brimming with tears. Recovery and rehabilitation collide. Progress is not easy. We will convene on this coming mid-October Thursday morning along with the rehab support crew, all due to this magnificent medical network this western world we live in affords us: physical therapist, occupational therapist, nurses, supplies and equipment, medications, procedures and protocols, a determined girl, wise yet not old, young. "Jackie is young," why she made it, why they invested so much in her. She could make it and did make it.

Jackie has plans and will begin launching them soon. She will figure it out. We will figure it out. We always do. Her dad and her brother, too.

A Writing About Mom from Dad

Well, Jackie will be home by Thursday. It is finally the end of the beginning of Jackie's new life. How sweet it is to hear and write those words. There is still much to do but Jackie will be in the capable hands, an understatement, of her mother. I, her father, will offer words of encouragement and watch movies with Jackie. The heavy lifting falls to her mother as it has for Jackie's life with cystic fibrosis. She truly is an amazing person. But that isn't surprising, her mother was one of the best people I have known. And her grandmother helped her grandfather run a farm, so it isn't surprising that she is able to care for Jackie as well as she does.

The great ones make it look easy but she has spent hours getting to know the intimate details of CF and learning what needs to be done and then doing it and doing it well. Tweak this, move that dial a little bit, add some of this, take away some of that. Always question, always move forward, trusting doctors but willing to challenge them if something doesn't seem right but always with graciousness and respect for their abilities and knowledge. There has been some pure luck in Jackie's life but most of the "luck" was created by Jackie's mom.

Journeying Back

Jackie became wickedly nauseated before the Thursday meeting, up most of the night, nauseated all the next day without reprieve and texted her transplant team. They attempted to adjust her medications from across town. Adam, the transplant pharmacist, works directly with patients. What he does is complicated and he gets it right, in part, by direct patient contact. Adam has been there all along, the right medications being so integral to transplant success. Jackie is transported back to Fairfax Hospital.

At the midnight hour, my exit is through the basement double doors by the emergency room. I happen upon a homeless woman, torn jeans not meant to be in style, moving upward to her worn face and distant eyes. "I'm so hungry. You got something I can eat?" I slide the baggie of cashews behind my hip and respond, "I don't." Maybe a different night but not this night. Someone else's turn.

I feel homeless myself wearing the same clothes for two, going on three days, what we do in times when changing clothes does not matter. What does matter is Jackie making it and making it back to her transplant team. They are the knowing ones, the willing ones, willing to take on this challenge, others in other fields willing to take on their own assigned challenges, a nice way to view the world we live in. We live in a world of the willing.

Jackie's medical transport through some unknown other exit is gone from here. I drive alone from that dark rehab parking lot in that dark place called, "Why?" Sweetwater Tavern crosses my mind. Jackie left, not by our car, not home with me to her dad, her dogs, her long-awaiting, freshly painted and ready bedroom. We are all ready. The question of the very young and innocent, the question, too, of the journeyers trying to get home, "Why?"

Jackie's intestines are acting up and rehab is not medical. She has to go back associated with her cystic fibrosis and gut problems, associated with her kidney dialysis and dehydration, associated with a most doable medical complexity that is Jackie's life. I have a few cross words for intestines, so lovable-hateable. They create nausea and vomiting or at least are willing participants. And nausea and vomiting create that timeless, endless feeling of awful. The brain and the intestines collude, as body systems sometimes do.

We can count on those body systems sorting it out. That's why for the most part, we're up and about, how Jackie will be when she gets past this unplanned side trip and gets fully home. Then she will be fully up and fully moving about within a few months, marked in my mind just past the last upcoming snowstorm. November, December, January... moving along into April, no snow, no ice, Jackie walking out to the car, Jackie going places. I can feel it in my brain tips.

Jackie feels relief in her intestines by way of that Fairfax Hospital magic of IV nutrition, IV medications, and a long, slow dose of bowel emptying solution most are familiar with for colonoscopy preps, oh dread. That hollow-eyed, ashen girl finally pinks up. The exhausting loop-de-loop ends with the tracheostomy also peeled away, free at last. Dr. Bobby steps in as many times before but this time, "You want it out?" Something that would have been so hard for so long, now so easy. Jackie and her lungs are ready, how sweet it is. Home, so close on this hard-fought journey, how sweet it will be. We don't need Sweetwater Tavern. Home will be escape enough.

Lest you think you live in a troubled country, take a look. Once again, that medical community does right and joyfully. We spend time looking at the Healing Garden through Jackie's hospital room window, the contents of her room reflecting in the glare but not for long. This room will be empty. I continue to scribble what crosses my mind each day and pull it together on posts each night. The comments back continue to be full of encouragement. It surely sustains us.

Brian

Brian and I went to high school together. In fact, we went to middle school together. I reached out to Brian when Jackie got so sick because I knew he cared and knew he knew others from way back who would care. I can look way back and assuredly know, his mother must have had fun raising Brian, so fortunate. Brian truly lives. He embraces the joys and challenges in days filled helping others in one legal bind or another, imaginable and unimaginable ones. Brian has his own set of stories. He's a defense attorney straddling between worlds of joy and worlds of sorrow as in any courtroom. It may be about being a lawyer but more about looking and seeing, knowing and helping.

He's successful in the real way because Brian is real. In high school, he sounded the morning PA announcements, pleasant and assured, grounding us each day, a nice place to be, a nice class of people to be with, Brian said it all and still does. I can hear that same sure voice in the courtroom, fortunate those who have him on their side. He doesn't win awards for no reason. Life as it should be, the fruits of a good life, living at potential, no sitting back.

Happy Jack is a lot like Brian, I like to think. When everyone is having a good time, multiply it. When something is fun, think "fun" and then some. Where does it come from, this intensity to live and live fully? Brian wrote on "Jackie's Get Well Update" post.

"I've only met you twice, enjoying dinner with your

family. Yet I love you with a joy that is real. Your mom is a good friend, and to read her posts is an ode to a mother's love that cannot easily be described. I'm part of "Team Jackie"—so many of us on this thread are—and it's a ride of ups and downs that we genuinely feel, but you experience. Sometimes totally aware, sometimes thankfully medicated into lala land. I think I speak for us all when I say we all cannot wait for you to re-start your "normal" life—at home, with friends, yes even at work. Please know that we're here. And we're never leaving you. Ever."

Brian shared with me a quote from Golden Globe winner Alex Ebert, "Even the most deft pen is a clumsy tool." It certainly is a deft tool describing the most joyful among us but when we see them, we know it.

This clumsy poem came to me.

live fully
joyful, spreading joy
happy, happy with the daily
living, truly living
focused, going places
real, no need to pinch themselves
life is fun, and thankful for it

Ebert's quote ends with, "...and yet we still try for magic." So true.

Alisa

～～～～～

I met Alisa on the phone when she asked if I could help with the Girl Scouts. I told her I wished I could but I was working full-time. She was working full-time. She was the Girl Scout leader. Jackie had countless well-spent adventuresome, all-things-creative hours with Emily at the Roman's house. Alisa wrote a poem, encouraging our family, this family of four, not three, four. Father, mother, brother... and sister.

"I am imagining Jackie
right up against a big wall...
it is a massive wall.
She is feeling anxious about it but she is climbing, ever so slowly,
with some slippage,
but there she goes.
During the climb,
with her nose pressed to the wall,
she can't see the gardens on the other side,
but she hangs on,
and soon she scoots over the top.
There,
there is the homecoming.
The celebratory,
healing sanctuary.
I am envisioning that.
Hang in there,

Jackie...and Jan, and Byron, and Byron,
and family and friends."
The garden on the other side... tomorrow.

We had so many thank yous, to Brian, to Alisa, to so many who saw us through and would continue to. Diane, just down the street, took care of our dogs. Her daughter, sweet Caroline, had created multiple childhood memories with Jackie with cookie dough and play dough and finger paint. Diane worked for years in an emergency room and moved to medical transport. She came to see Jackie every week, understanding the difficult and able to explain progress. She talked to me late at night, stopped by our house early in the morning, brought meals, brought a smile, brought hope, and we were grateful.

Jackie was liberated from her tracheostomy in Fairfax Hospital on October 16 with assurance that her new lungs would breathe and breathe without back up. Dr. Bobby always said it would happen and we believed him, and it did happen. Five days to go by then, five days of life still in Heart and Vascular Institute but not in the ICU. The Acute Pulmonary Unit nurse-patient ratio was not one-on-one or one-on two, but one-on-five, closer to where a patient would want to be, closer to going home back to conversations with her father at our kitchen table.

Her Dad Writes About Doubts

I wish I could say I had no doubts; the first few weeks were brutal, as our son said. Jackie's mother always thought she would make it. What a roller coaster it was for the first couple of months. All I can say is thank you to all the people who have been indispensable in her return to kith and kin. I could have gone my whole life being ignorant about things like ECMO and been quite content but maybe that isn't a good thing.

I have been able to witness firsthand the tremendous goodness of people, the remarkable inventions we humans are capable of and how great the body of knowledge there must be to have facilitated her return. I am truly amazed by what I have witnessed over the last four months: the focused mental and physical effort that so many people have exerted to save Jackie's life and return her to the world. I am so grateful in so many ways.

Jackie: Home!

I've waited 136 long days for today. The battle I didn't even know I would be fighting started on June 10 and today, I am finally home. The hardest 136 days of my life, some of which I have no memory of, a faded memory of, or am told by my family.

I sit here and take deep breaths and can feel my lungs fill all the way with air, no more constant coughing. I am breathing easy and in the comfort of my own home. My legs are still weak so my wheeler (walker with wheels) and I are still good friends. The next few weeks will be filled with doctor appointments, dialysis, and physical therapy. I am hoping to get stronger every day and get back my independence.

I call the group of doctors that saved my life "My Team." My Team also includes Lauren, an inpatient nurse practitioner who knows her stuff, and sees me through. Leaving the hospital means leaving her care. I am ready for the "outpatient" nurse practitioners. Still it's a hard break from Lauren.

My Team came in today to send me off and I shed a few tears thanking them and telling them I thought I would never see today. Although, at first, there were doubts that I was going to make it, they knew I was strong and had a will to survive. I can never thank them enough. All I have to say is Fairfax Hospital is the best place with the greatest doctors, nurses, respiratory therapists and physical/occupational therapists.

I can't forget about my donor. Today I told my parents I couldn't believe someone else's lungs were in me. My dad said, "They're your lungs now." They're my lungs now and they're healthy. Although they are my lungs now, I will never forget the family that donated their loved one's organs. I owe them my life. I hope next year they are willing to meet me but at the very least I will send them a letter of gratitude.

The act of organ donation will save someone's life as it did mine, and I encourage everyone to become one. If not an organ donor, donate your body to science to help fight disease and find cures.

Now to sleep in my own bed...

Eventful

The ride home, uneventful, Jackie and mom in the car riding away from the outside fountain, after taking the elevator down, passing the inside fountain, the ride home along the well-worn path, quiet conversation, as always. Pulling up to our house, a simple sign on the door, "Welcome home, Jackie." Jackie's steps are slow, assisted by a walker and a mom.

Once she reaches the threshold, she speeds clumsily down the home hallway, down the home office hallway to a chair by her father and collapses in an eruption of tears. Weeks upon weeks of emotion seep from every pore, fear and sorrow, patience and long-suffering, anxiety and anticipation, hope and joy, and there with her father again, at home again. She almost tries to get up and walk to him, forgetting that she cannot get up and walk, as if the lapse of the past months weren't. Home, peaceful, eventful.

What seemed like well in the hospital seems like sick at home. Reality. Jackie has to be careful. I have to be helpful. Some of the medications that help her cope with anxiety and sleeplessness associated with serious hospital stays are pulled back; neuropathic pain shimmers down her body. I hold her tight with all my might one night, getting her through to morning when she makes a new plan, to slowly pull back on those medications, which Jackie successfully will but in her own way in her own time.

This is the Jackie they knew they were transplanting, interactive and responsible. We'll deal with what comes, being hot, being cold, hungry, annoyed, the itchy feet, cramping legs, "Hurry, I don't want to be alone," "Go away and leave me alone." Yet this is still the Jackie I know, persistent and hope-filled.

The scars will heal, from chest tubes and ECMO twice, from intestinal surgery and laparoscopic surgery, from swelling and blistering, so many scars. What a symphony, certainly not music to Jackie's ears. Each of her scars, I remind her, represents someone's efforts to save her life, someone who took the time to develop those skills and to apply them when called upon in the most horrific of circumstances. So many different names and faces, so many different personalities, its own symphony, certainly music to our ears.

Her father comes upon our conversation, a pause putting thoughts together, an interjection. "Jackie, who you are is from the neck up. What's important is what's between your ears. Your body will heal. Take care of your body and allow it to take care of itself over time. Focus on what's important and that's from the neck up." Jackie has always done well from the neck up. She listens.

In college, there was a rash of break-ins so I appealed to Jackie not to stay alone in her townhouse if her roommates were away, and one night they were away. We received a 2 a.m. landline call from the Radford police saying there was a break-in and they only found Jackie's wallet. Was she drunk and committing crimes with fellow college drunks? I scrambled to call Jackie's cell phone from my cell phone as the officer hung up, "The parent isn't cooperating."

I then scrambled to call the Radford dispatcher who confirmed the authenticity of the call and location, Jackie's townhouse. She had been kidnapped. I made nightmarish calls to her brother, her dad and I wired out the rest of the night. In the morning, Jackie called. Her phone had been off. She had been asleep. She had just learned of the break-in, front door frame nearly torn off. The noise must have prompted neighbors to call the police. No wallet was stolen. Jackie's wallet had been left by the police, by the robbers who fled, and by Jackie who had left to spend the night with a friend rather than stay alone that night in that townhouse. She had listened.

Our son had listened, as well, and was in a sweet spot in the science world. Seeking a grant from the National Science Foundation, he wrote, "Time flows, time flies, time heals. You can save time, lose time, find time, race against time. Some people hit the big time, other have a bad time. What a mess! Thankfully, physics provides some clarity in all of the chaos." The hope in neuroscience, he explained to us, is to build more accurate artificial networks that mimic the brain, brain models that will learn in real time, be flexible, and interact with their environment. Byron would like to research changes in the brain over time not associated with aging. "The human brain self-organizes allowing us to learn."

When I asked Jackie's dad to summarize for us what Byron's National Science Foundation application statement was about, he said it was beyond him though I think not. Her brother concluded, "Our goal is to become better shepherds of ourselves, body and mind, and our environment." Being home meant Jackie shepherding her own care. She was getting well and though complicated, by the hour, for Jackie, her care was not complicated. I continued to update weekly as Jackie herself began to write more regularly.

Post-transplant care proved to be an avalanche of biometrics both at home and at the Inova Advanced Lung Disease and Transplant clinic: monitoring the pulse, the oxygen, the lung capacity, temperature, blood pressure, blood sugar, blood chemistry. Did I leave anything out? I'd look at

Jackie in all of this. She was home, she was real, and she was Jackie. We got our way in a big way.

Redefined

Still so many stories like the little girl at the store who asks the big girl why she is wearing a mask and what she will be for Halloween. The people who know most why Jackie is wearing a mask are the transplant team members who see her twice a week, the people at the dialysis center who see her three times a week still aiming for the kidneys to come back because a kidney transplant would not be a story we would want to tell. The store, the new lungs, the use of their battery-packed people cart with the food basket up front plus the not-far walking ignite Jackie to buy far too much food, much anticipation fulfilled.

I begin to think how successful we are in life depends on our ability to redefine ourselves. "I walked away from a big university almost before I started." "I'm no longer loved by my husband." "I now have an only child." "I don't have my own lungs anymore." How do we redefine ourselves? What allows us to? Strength and resilience? That we have no choice? Or do we have a choice? Remain evermore centered on what was, is no more, can't be, going through the motions holding on anyhow or letting go of what was, shifting on that path?

"I'm someone who can't walk anymore and live well in my head." "I became wealthy yet kept my feet planted firmly on the ground." "I came out of drug rehab after a family intervention. Yes, that's me."

"I'm the girl at twenty-five who has new lungs and a story that's long and hard."

Resilience is different from loss. Loss causes that inescapable stark hollow rod of pain within. Resilience helps us deal with it. Resilience means redefining ourselves. There must be some organic reworking that allows us to survive loss, to be resilient. It's messy but then life is messy and we seek to tidy it up like that ICU tidied up Jackie's life and now she will make her own way. She will redefine herself.

CHAPTER EIGHT

NOVEMBER SLIPPED IN

I picked up the phone one morning in early November, just two weeks home, and dialed the ENT, the ear, nose, and throat specialist who operated on Jackie right before her lungs went down. "I'm calling to make an appointment for Jacqueline Price." "What type of appointment does she need?" "Follow up to sinus surgery." She didn't know and didn't need to know. It was as if those past five months hadn't happened but they had happened. I thought back.

We stepped back and allowed them to do what they do best, and they did. There was no fault-finding. There was no begging God. Steady and quiet intentions we placed before God and man and we made our way home following up, those transplanted lungs working well. Jackie seated on the couch with no more coughing because no more cystic fibrosis lungs was amazing and home was where I wanted her to stay.

Jackie wanted to go out but not stay out and not drink.

She had experienced something quite different from everybody else at the party. She was wearing a mask. She was not the same because she had lived through a major medical event with a difficult recovery at a young age.

What had not changed was Jackie's singular focus on working in her field of finance, returning part-time to her job when the recovery time was right. She'd been to dinner with friends and to lunch with co-workers, people and food. She was walking more, gaining strength, still going to dialysis, still wearing that one pair of slippers over swollen feet, and still planning on wearing those long-awaited shoes. Jackie was making that shift.

I, too, was making a shift, viewing life as story. Every day, what I thought and felt, experienced and witnessed, I captured in thought and sometimes in scribble and writing. What I wrote before, what I will write to come, melds together into one long story broken up by characters and events and portions of life that make up the whole. Creativity has a way of gaining on itself. I grew excited at the thought.

Creative Christine was a big part of our update group, cheering Jackie on and continuing to through art. She is an artist who drew and posted beautiful abstract pen and watercolors of shoes representing Jackie's love of shoes. Christine came over to share her creativity with Jackie. I heard laughter and instruction in the other room as they forged a friendship and Jackie grew to love art. There's a cushioned, comfortable chair situated at an art table by the shelving full of pens and markers, sponges and brushes, rainbows of color for hours of "Zentangles."

Jackie had time for art between medical appointments and a cut-back on dialysis days, time while waiting for swelling to go down, for shoes and boots to fit. She had time for physical therapists to come to our house and join the wide range of special people who help others for a living. Maybe we all help each other for a living. Maybe time was all that was important, each moment of each day in some way, helping each other.

Time

Time... the truth teller, the healer, the gift
Time allows time to sort it all out
What happened?
It would've been called suffering
But it's more a chance to be happy again
To smile with friends, hug family
Do art, play games, follow the news
To think and dream and worry
And hum or whistle, to shrug and nod and doze
To feel, beautiful skin, slender dainty fingers
Feet that tickle, back that itches
To open curtains to the morning sunshine
And close them to night darkness looking out on
what unknown
To be real, to feel, to know
that only time takes away pain
Brings new life to a well led life
Time brings strength, recovery, wellness
Time... the truth teller, the healer, the gift.

We're Back

"No acute rejection," words sweet to embrace after a biopsy just before Thanksgiving under general anesthesia by Dr. Bobby at Fairfax Hospital, the not-so-long-ago place we called home. Getting on the elevator isn't about that absence-of-mind-rush-in like before. Down, not up, to Pulmonary Rehab, the place to go when moving on.

The anesthesiologist, not the first engineer-turned-doctor we'd met, laughs that his parents paid for his education so he then decided to go to medical school. I'm sure they appreciated his smarts. He introduces himself before the procedure as usual, but this time, "Hi, I know you well even though you don't know me. I worked a lot in June and you had quite a busy month." I wonder what it is like for him seeing this smiling young girl after seeing her over and again in that June quagmire.

There are lots of smiles in that pulmonary procedure area today. Hundreds of hours of medical preparation converging upon the girl who made it and here she is. "Where'd the scars on your neck come from?" one unknowing nurse asks. She listens, she hesitates, she speaks, "You're a special person." Yea, we're all special. I get that. I'd like to be special. I think and look over at my smiling daughter enjoying this arena of people she is now an insider with. Yea, she's special. Yea, I'm thankful. "No acute rejection." Cooking with friends, drawing with pens and such, pulling out the winter coats, getting a new haircut. Yea, special. Every day, special.

Thankful

~~~~~~~~

Thankful top to bottom

Inside out and upside down

Back and forth

Over and under

This way and that

Thankful

Food was always a big part of our family, my sister always reminded me. The four of us, Byron, Byron, Jan, and Jackie, always conjured up feasts and carried them through. Both Byron and Jackie had at points as adults moved back home and both had received comments about improved look of health, their mother must have been feeding them. One was from a teacher Byron worked with, the other Dr. Brown to Jackie. I took those as high compliments as I read through my cookbooks, pleasure reading when time wasn't so short.

Anne and I always agreed that if I cooked, she would clean up and she gladly always did. This year, I did not want to cook Thanksgiving dinner. I wanted to rest. Jackie wanted to eat and someone who was steady on their feet had to cook and that would not be Jackie. Her eating had outrun her walking, sometimes a meal just before or after a meal. We delighted in fattening those little fingers up. So her brother, Byron, and her cousin, Joshua, cooked. I highly recommend twenty-something guys making the Thanksgiving meal. Every pan in the kitchen got dirty but Jackie was eating heartily by then and my sister and I thankfully cleaned up together.

CHAPTER NINE

AND THEN IT WAS DECEMBER

December arrived and we had adapted our lives around the demands. Jackie's dad had help in his home office. He and I half-connected as I whiplashed through each and every day helping Jackie stay safe and on track getting where she needed to go. The house was reorganized with a cushioned living room chair placed at the end of the kitchen table, a new couch placed in the living room meeting the physical demands of a boney young lady trying to gain weight. Food was central and meals were hearty and healthy and yummy. Jackie ate and slept and planned her life. I planned the linen closet.

Life in the Linen Closet

~~~~~~~~

How many times do you have to get out of the shower and no towel, race to the linen closet, cold and wet, hope the curtains are closed, before you realize that linens don't belong in the linen closet? When we cleared the linen closet to dedicate it to Jackie's medical care, I put the towels nicely in the bathrooms, and tucked the sheets away in drawers near the beds. Vavoom! Linen closets are not meant for linens. Art supplies, yes. Wine, maybe. Anything emblematic or thematic and preferably fun. If you have already rededicated your linen closet, I'm late to the party... again.

Here's Jackie's transplant life in the linen closet, shelf by shelf...

Pill bottles, twenty-something of them in a bin

Nebulizers, we hope to never use again

Syringes, all sizes for pushing fluids and getting medications in

Squirt bottle, antibiotics, and saline for sinus irrigation

Antibiotic ointment, wound dressing, anti-flu suspension

More syringes, insulin

Protein powder, calorie sprinkle, nutrition shakes

Alcohol preps, q-tips, and the gauze it takes

Hospital tape and hospital tape

Night nutrition, supplemental food

Cans and bags and a connector tube

Enzyme cartridges that are new

(Thank you to Blue Cross/Blue Shield!)

Life couldn't be all about writing poems about linen closets. Life was also about worry, and worry, her father and I did.

Worry

I'm trying to figure out "worry" and figure it out from my own mind, untarnished by experts. Leaving an ICU with a daughter with newly transplanted lungs is a worry. Right when our daughter is putting the enormity of an ICU stay behind her, the kidney transplant teamers show up to talk to her. Making it through the ICU made a lung transplant less of a worry but a lung transplant makes a kidney transplant still a worry. But then the kidney doctors say a kidney transplant is less of a worry because of the lung transplant, same drugs, same routine, much easier surgery.

This is like playing hide-and-seek with the worry bully, the one up there hanging around in my head. Like with any bully, I can ignore it, humor it, join it, let it get to me, let it not get to me. Maybe "worry" finds its comfortable place up there and settles in and is not "worry" anymore. It becomes a part of who I am and doesn't act out so much. The bully becomes a companion of sorts. So today maybe we're okay that we don't know if Jackie will need a kidney transplant. She's going to dialysis twice a week and two of my book group friends, Mary and Chris, are taking turns bringing her home, giving Jackie a break from her worrisome mother.

Another friend is taking a trip to Ireland this week and I told her we're taking a trip, too, to the dialysis center. The dialysis center is its own trip. Seeing people with missing feet reminds me to worry less. I guess worry and proper perspective run on the same playground. Enjoying the very sound of our daughter's voice, appreciating her fingers flying across those cell phone keys, viewing her beautiful Zentangle creations, hearing her laugh with friends makes worry silly.

Now that I think about it, that I am not in a constant state of heightened worry must mean that I'm not much of a worrier after all, so I think I'll leave the figuring out to the experts. Just as I always believed Jackie would come home again, I believe Jackie will not need a kidney transplant. And Jackie does not seem so worried herself so I'll take her advice. "Calm down, mom."

The name of the game was always to keep Jackie out of the hospital. The thought cringed the veins my blood ran through or at least I imagined it cringed them. My friend, Mona, used to work downtown in a high-stress job and when I'd ask her how she was doing, on occasion she would say, "Shattered, just shattered." With her beautiful Egyptian accent, she would say more like, "Shatta-ed, just shatta-ed." Mona knew Jackie from when she was a small child and when she came to see Jackie in the hospital, I think it did nearly shatter Mona. That's how we felt one night just before Christmas. But then, we were not shattered.

A Night

If you've ever had a colonoscopy, you've ingested this creepy bowel-emptying substance. Preparation for that procedure is regrettable. If you develop a bowel obstruction, you may slowly ingest this stuff under medical supervision to gently erupt and resolve the obstruction.

If you develop a bowel obstruction, you are very sick and the seriousness can escalate but once resolved, you are well again. Cystic fibrosis, known as mucoviscidosis in Europe, sticky mucus disease, not always compatible with smooth bowel action. Jackie's new lungs do not have cystic fibrosis and they are doing well. Her gut still does and is doing well due to a now widely used over-the-counter somewhat scaled back version of the "bowel prep" solution.

We don't know why, maybe the timing of taking her gut medications was off, but she was doing very well yesterday and last night at two in the morning woke up with a bowel obstruction, two wicked awful lumps of pain in her abdomen, doubled-over-in-pain kind of pain. So we pulled out the solution and since Jackie has the g-tube, that silicone valve access to her stomach on her abdomen, we slow-dripped it in. No resolution so with a white knuckled grip, I dialed the on-call transplant line and of course, we had to go to the emergency room.

I called my sister by three in the morning to come help, and began to pull Jackie's belongings together to take her to the hospital. "Turn it up!" Jackie said. "Turn the rate up!" "What?" I'm thinking.

"I am not going to the hospital, turn the rate up!" Jackie knows her gut and she knows it well and she knew she could handle more so I turned the rate up on the pump. My sister and I lay across Jackie's bed as she lay there in pain but not so much pain that she could not talk, yet those awful wads in her intestines held on. Our aversion to going to the emergency room held on.

We all three began to doze. Jackie fell sound asleep. We stirred and slipped out to other bedrooms and all slept until morning. We are still home, not at the hospital, and Jackie's belly is soft. She rid her own self of that blockage-forming poop.

Dr. King contacted Jackie, having been told when he came into the hospital in the morning that Jackie was in the emergency room, yet she was not. The blockage passed and we will spend today emotionally recuperating and then get more of that creepy medicine to keep in the linen closet. This stuff has kept many people out of the hospital and if we stay on top of the daily dosing, we believe it will continue to keep Jackie out of the hospital.

Jackie wrote online about her life-saving, emergency bi-lateral lung transplant, how it turned her life upside down, how she expected to be in the hospital less than a week returning to work in the immediate. Instead, in the immediate she was texting friends that she was scared, that she did not know what was going to happen, that she loved them and thanked them for being such great friends in those hours before coma and intubation. This was the worst experience in her life but in some strange way, the best. She wrote about her lungs, no longer with disease, no longer that constant cough, her plan to run again, to honor her donor. We anticipated a lot of demands post-transplant but we did not anticipate the complex maze of recovery. It would not spoil our gratitude.

Christmas was peaceful with Jackie's brother home and lots of gift giving, eating and relaxing, life as it should be. Rejection was on our minds throughout the Christmas season. Jackie's friend, Jason, experienced a lung transplant a few years ago and experienced a good after-transplant life married to a beautiful wife, working as a paramedic. Jason was someone I reached out to first when Jackie was on ECMO. He has a way of knowing what a fighter Jackie is because he is a fighter.

Jason's lungs went down. His last text to Jackie, "It's my turn now. I'm heading to Duke." That was all he wrote and all he needed to write. His transplant had been at Duke University Hospital and his recovery this time, avoiding a second transplant, was at Duke University Hospital. ECMO, that maybe-life-saving lung machine, saved Jason's life. Like Jackie, many cherishable lives reside in one cherishable person.

Throughout the holiday season, Jackie practiced walking up and down the hallway of our house without her walker. She was wobbly at first, grabbing the wall every now and then but every day, she felt less like she was going to fall. On Christmas Eve, we delivered cookies to the wonderful nurses of the CVICU who had to work during the holiday. It was a family affair. Jackie decided to leave her walker at the entrance and later wrote about it.

Jackie: Calming

I saw one of my favorite nurses and walked up to her. She couldn't believe it. One nurse, Audrey, a charge nurse for a lot of my stay, came up a little later. I was sitting when she saw me so I got up again, walked over and gave her a hug. She told me with tears in her eyes there was a reason I survived, I had a meaning in life and there were big plans for me. That felt calming and wonderful to hear. I was also told that I had been their greatest success story of 2016. Those doctors & nurses worked so hard, they're my biggest success story of 2016.

CHAPTER TEN

JANUARY MEANT A
PROMISING NEW YEAR

Getting rid of the walker became the focus. On New Year's Eve, Jackie and her friends had a reservation at a chic restaurant in nearby Arlington, followed by a party in a rented game room on the top floor of an apartment building. It was low- keyed and unhurried, so Jackie went to both without her walker. So tired and wanting to call for a ride home, Jackie with friends pushed for the well-deserved ringing in of the New Year as the Times Square ball on the screen dropped.

We went to the hospital the next week to get labs drawn at Outpatient, left the walker in the car in the garage, then realized Jackie didn't need it but as a seat to rest on for long distances. The first week of January, six months by then since the take-down, Jackie could officially walk again, admittedly with an odd limp caused by very tight hip muscles and further need for physical therapy.

Ridding the walker and being in Outpatient were not

the only milestones met. What a stark contrast to those In-patient days. Jackie could get up from a seat without help. She could walk up stairs while spotted, and do laundry. Most of her shoes fit, so no more slipper wearing out in public. Her lung functions were up to 45% and rising and she had memorized all of her medication names and doses filling her 4x7 compartmentalized pillbox with dozens of those various little shapes. These milestones might be taken for granted by those unknowing ones around us as Jackie's medical condition grew more invisible.

Her brother remained in town into the first of the year and he took Jackie to medical appointments, social engagements, and shopping malls. Jackie could make it through an entire evening "in DC" but among the happy times were times of darkness. Jackie remained in bed in a curtain-drawn room for a couple of days and we took the risk of going out to dinner without her. She normally did not like to stay alone in our house at night as we live in the woods down a country road.

We drove that twenty minutes to a nice restaurant after much deliberation, Jackie telling us to leave her alone. She'd done well thus far and she would work this through and continue to do well both mentally and physically. Fortunately for Jackie and for us, the next day two of her sorority sisters, held dear, brought a beautiful purple bracelet band inscribed, "Always Brave." The attached card read, "Falling down is a part of life. Getting back up is living." Jackie began to peel away thoughts of wanting her former life back, replaced by thoughts of her new life.

Jackie's To Do List

Goals.

Do art.

Ride the stationary bike.

End dialysis without needing a kidney transplant.

Go back to work by summer.

Stand from a seated position on the floor.

Gain some good abs!

Pray to God for Jason.

Get the shoes on to get to lots of places.

Shoes

Today has been a stressful day. Where do we put fifty pairs of shoes in a not very large bedroom? Not meaning to kiss and tell but the exact count is fifty-four pairs of shoes and maybe even another by the front door. I'm afraid to look. Some shoes, we removed already, those spike-heeled ones that would aggravate the neuropathy that had calmed down in Jackie's feet. Some shoes are too narrow as Jackie tried them all on today. Maybe her feet have changed. Maybe Jackie has changed.

I frequently look over and can't believe Jackie is sitting there. She's still funny and fun and gets annoyed, then gets over it. She's ten pounds less than when she got so sick in June rather than the twenty pounds less just a bit ago. Her voice has not returned to full range after those weeks of intubation and maybe it won't according to the speech therapist at the hospital. Metal and plastic and throats don't do too well together but well enough to save lives. I always thought intubation meant "that's it" but those folks apparently pop those things in and out of people all the time and it's not necessarily "It," thank heavens.

Jackie has a nice voice with a quirky twist... raising her voice lowers her volume. Jackie can't yell. She's not a yeller anyhow. She doesn't need to yell. Her dad calls her "Attila the Honey" and always has. She walks with a slight waddle and better not get bumped into. She's slight and slightly off balance yet ditched the walker, a bragging right we couldn't have made up. But yes, and yesterday, someone questioned why she needed access to the elevator when patrons use the stairs.

Apparently Jackie is shedding her hospital patient look. She wears the germ exchange prevention mask but not every waking minute she's out. As long as no one sprays their germy spit on her since her anti-rejection drugs will anti-reject colds and flus and viruses, as well. We have to get through winter without that going on. Good hand sanitizing, be careful not to go from germy surfaces to face. Ick! Germs are spread most readily from direct spew, not clear across the room, according to Adam, the transplant pharmacist who then has to determine what drugs to give to shoo off those nasty causers of sickness.

Jackie's going out when times are too special to miss, which means every chance to be with friends but then she's home and wants the house temperature set at eighty degrees. She's still fragile and can't sit on the floor then get up, so I'm helping her organize those shoes in shoe holders and we're getting along well for a mom who was going to launch into "the kids are gone" and a daughter who was going to launch into "I don't live at home anymore." Jackie plans, Lord willing (and the Lord certainly has been willing), to drive soon when her legs and reflexes are stronger and eventually not live at home anymore when she's much, much stronger. She'll be taking those shoes with her.

She reached a low point over the holidays, a brief launch reversal but we always work it out around here. It's a loving home and Jackie's reclaiming her life bit by bit in the warmth. Some of the shoes need stretchers, it seems, so like everything and everyone around here, we'll keep pushing and pulling and tugging and stretching and getting through stressful and not as stressful days. The girl has much to do and those shoes are waiting no more.

CHAPTER ELEVEN

MIXED NEWS DEFINED FEBRUARY

The skies in winter in our area are often overcast but they would not cast a shadow on my mind, or Jackie's, no matter the news, good or bad. The dialysis catheter was removed and the need for dialysis, yet we still attended a multi-hour kidney transplant appointment to cover the ever-present future possibility. The kidneys did make it back, beating well-established statistics, timeframes after which the kidneys aren't likely to come back. Jackie went outside that timeframe by months. For her in the moment, this meant taking a shower without protecting an access attached to the body that couldn't get wet. We were used to using layers of plastic wrap and tape but never got that part near water, so Jackie never bathed without caution and help until this good news.

Then the bad news: fever and possible pneumonia threw Jackie back into the hospital, creating another access to the body for more medications and in the moment, another delay on a shower. Maybe Jackie had aspirated, coughed and a small piece of something went down the wrong pipe, or her still-cystic fibrosis sinuses were dripping the tiniest of nasties down to her lungs. Immunosuppressant drugs could be inviting infection. They would figure it out again.

Once the laboratory determined what bug was getting after her, they matched it head-to-head with IV antibiotics and Jackie went home again. She waited seven months to take a real shower or a real bath, her choice. Dreams of a bubble bath popped, a couple more weeks of waiting.

The "dread" of winter was not full of snow and ice and we were thankful for no icy patches, falls or injuries. Jackie demanded good food from our kitchen and demanded that we work on this 2000-piece puzzle, Cinque Terra, a puzzle of five small rocky seaside villages located in Italy. We wish we were there, so beautiful. Instead, we were here, so beautiful.

Jackie and her dad put bets out that I would crumble at some point and they laughed about it. When Byron was home from Boston, he pointed out the possibility that they forego that one bottle of barbecue sauce if it meant mom having to get up again. We orchestrated well enough the care of everyone in the house and some days, there were clashes. Dad needed me, Jackie needed me, the bacon on the stove needed me! Dad learned if he said Jackie needed it, even if she didn't need it and he did, I would get it. And I would. I would get anything for Jackie and anything for her dad only sometimes!

Each day was like putting puzzle pieces together, successfully navigating all the demands of care. My son had said, "Mom, you won't be able to do it." I thought about the mom of a student I once had. Walking toward the grocery line after school one day, I looked up and saw her with that deer-in-the-headlights look, eyes darting about as if in near-captivity. Her children were prone to attempts at jumping out of moving cars with no father to catch them. I never wanted to look like that and made sure I didn't. Hearing singing or whistling down the hallway helped, Jackie like old times.

Recovery

Recovery, fast-paced yet slow, like so many human processes, like learning, packed days in the long slow process of twelve years, more like thirteen years and that's just getting started. I often think about all the doctors we encountered, all we have gotten to know, and are yet to meet. Dr. Adam Pearlman was there and he knew and he said Jackie and I were remarkable. We needed to hear that. Thanks to Dr. Pearlman for his kind words back when we were low, seeking his understanding to settle our understanding of ICU pain and swelling and immobility, and now oh sweet recovery.

Dr. Pearlman, precise and thorough, went over with us all of Jackie's blood work numbers at the nephrology appointment. This number is up, that one is down, some matter, some don't, some matter but lungs matter more. Jackie's kidneys are still complicated, and still cooperating. He and his partners will keep an eye on Jackie's numbers from her pulmonary appointment blood draws. Those labs are too important to slip by nephrology. Who would have thought we would need nephrology?

Who would have thought we would need dermatology? Those tiny dark buggers we haul around on our skin could mean trouble due to those lovable anti-rejection drugs. We would be foolish not to add dermatology to the appointment calendar. We run here and run there allowing those people who finished grade twelve and then did twelve more to tell people like us what to do. That's recovery.

Behind the Scenes

A lot goes on behind the scenes to keep those lungs breathing. Jackie's dad always believes in the "rule of threes" and my understanding of Jackie's lung care does come in threes. First, the immunosuppressive drugs inhibit the immune response that would reject the lungs, the balance maintained by drawing blood, testing levels, and adjusting medication dosages, done weekly or more, then biweekly, then less frequently over time. The immunosuppression welcomes the new lungs, and welcomes infection, thus the constant hand washing and occasional mask wearing but that's not enough.

Second, "IVIG" infusions, immune-strengthening immunoglobulin, elements of blood made available by blood plasma donors, infused monthly for Jackie. The immune system is both suppressed and brought back to strength by the balance of all these drugs in order to fight infection and that brings the third, white blood count.

White blood cells make up just one percent of the blood, one white blood cell for every four hundred

red blood cells but they are not to be taken lightly. When white blood cell counts go up, they are fighting infection. When they go down, infection is fighting the body, and winning. A good guess would be, yes, another medication given to increase the white blood count by demanding more from the beloved bone marrow we all take for granted. This medication, given as needed based on healthy white blood count, ranges based on blood work, blood work being the essential link to the success of transplant. And three is enough for me!

Our online updates slowed down. Jackie ran around town on her own by then, going to physical therapy twice a week and to a professional football training facility twice a week. Cory worked at this gym unlike any gym concept we'd experienced and volunteered during off hours to help Jackie regain strength and stamina. The place was empty except an occasional athlete would pass by Jackie, twice her size, bench-pressing twice her weight as she lifted but five pounds. At that, her lung function went up above 50%, the highest since the year 2010. In spite of the fever-IV antibiotic hiccup of a hospital stay, she was enjoying life with her new lungs. Her necklace read, "Breathe." I wanted a necklace that read, "Breathe, appreciate, breathe."

CHAPTER TWELVE

MARCH BROUGHT ANTICIPATION

The March winds might have been blowing but Jackie's lungs were calm, no infection and no rejection determined at her nine-month bronchoscopy. The next bronchoscopy would be at the one-year "lungiversary." With that good news, Jackie submitted paperwork to return to work in the spring, eight hours per week to start, to get back to Lidl. Jackie got out to enjoy wineries without the wine, and rooftop restaurants in the District of Columbia. And then there were rest and recuperate days, staying hydrated, avoiding food-borne and air-borne illnesses.

Then, a fever arose and another hospitalization. First year of transplants are like that. Jackie, with a 103-degree fever and a feverish swollen area at the top of her now shapely leg, began throwing up. Thank God for kind nurses. Those lungs were clear and Jackie presented well. Was this a wave, not a tidal wave, maybe even a splash?

Jackie had a patch of cellulitis easily receding with a little

IV potion and she went home in three days, intravenous line-free. Even though they are able to poke people with needles and tubules and daggers and then slip curatives in and send them home with the home IV entourage, this time home without it was a relief. I reminded Jackie, again, she would be home and have gained her independence from all of this by the last possible snowfall and it would somehow be so.

Jackie missed no beat returning to the pro-football gym with Cody. There's always a vignette behind the vignette. When Jackie showed her father a video clip of her pushing an athlete training sleigh across the empty gym floor, he responded, "You don't get a trophy for showing up." Jackie's response, "My dad's an ass." He first wanted to know how much weight it was in order to factor in the frictional coefficient. Besides coming home to her wonderful dad, Jackie wanted to come home to a wonderful dog. Oh great, something else to take care of. At least the warmer weather would arrive before getting the dog.

The Dog

Soon after Jackie came home from the hospital, she determined that taking care of herself was not enough. Jackie needed someone else to take care of, so she stole my miniature Dachshund from me. But wait, Frank was hers. But wait again. Then seventh grade Jackie brought her new baby Dachshund home at 4 p.m. and by 8 a.m. the next morning wanted nothing to do with Frank so Frank and his two-year potty training escapade became mine. Indeed, Frank is mine and Frank is a crazy lovable bandit of a dog.

I took a gamble and told Jackie this time before getting a dog, she would need to run it by her transplant team. Of course, these doctors have no problem saying "no" but in this case, they said "yes." (Imagine running everything by a team of smart-minded adults running your life… buying a plane ticket, joining an exercise program, getting a dog.) Apparently they are strict and flexible. Eeek!

At the same time, a show dog of the Madison Square Garden Westminster Kennel Club variety, wow that is, lost sight in one eye, lost the eye. Maybe Westminster should have their own form of Special Olympics but for now, one-eyed, seven-and-a-half pound, hairless Chinese crested Fae needed Jackie and Jackie needed her, today being the day. My friend Lynn and her daughter Jamie, dog trainers extraordinaire, brought Fae to Jackie and will mentor Jackie in being the reciprocal companion of this three-year-old show dog now turned beloved pet. It's as if Fae has been here all along. It's as if we were thankful all along.

CHAPTER THIRTEEN

SPRINGTIME ALREADY

Jackie remained fully capable of handling her affairs, medical and personal, responding in the negative to a call for jury duty, researching viable health insurance options for when she turned twenty-six, reading articles written about what happened to her, planning an upcoming speaking event, and stepping further back into her social life. With all this going on, this girl had an amazing disposition.

Disposition

Disposition. Dictionary definitions combined say, "the prevailing tendency of one's spirit, quality of mind and character, mental and emotional outlook or mood." I love a good disposition. For me, being around someone with a good disposition is like the first day of spring, every time. It's good for the soul.

I would like to have a good disposition but life circumstances perhaps have made me more of a street fighter, a bit roughed up around the edges and I can't seem to do anything about that.

In our update group is a teacher friend I worked with for years. I loved her gentle disposition and so did her students. Her nature was inherently easy, I thought, until I met her sister who joined our teaching staff and she also had that beautiful disposition, predictably kind, taking each day as it came, unruffled by the goings on. Their father (mother having passed away) was a big part of their lives and I wanted to meet him just in time for parenting disposition lessons to learn how to teach my own children to have that good way about them, never stirring up something or other, yet not getting pushed around. Easy. Pulling it off. At the end of each school day, Peggy and Lynn were people we were glad to have spent the day with, always part of the solution with a gentle smile. Our principal, instead, used to say to me, "What have you done now?"

Once, a mom, who tried to keep her second-grader home too much stopped by to check him out of school again, came to my classroom door. I stepped out to ask why. She said a family member had died. I said, "I want to know who died." When she told me, actually a friend of hers, "You're not taking him out" escaped from my mouth. She left. I avoided our principal.

Even still, I am sure my own children were impacted by the disposition recognition and I am sure our home was better for it. Peggy has encouraged Jackie in her recovery like so many and we are grateful and can't ever loop back to say thank you enough, yet it is so.

Enter Pam. Her son has cystic fibrosis and we've been friends since coming together as a group of parents of young children with this disease trying to figure out what now, what next, what. I always know how Pam will be. Pam removes so many complications in life. What an impact on the lives around her. Pam spent time with Jackie last time in the hospital when I couldn't be there. So good for Jackie. Pam makes quilts... thematic quilts, clever and colorful quilts... for people when they retire or their dog dies, when they suffer or celebrate, Pam buried in her downstairs sewing room spreading her goodness. Yes, Jackie got a quilt in her favorite colors and "thank you" is not enough for the quilt or for the wonderfulness of Pam's disposition.

Enter Fae. Are dogs born this way or does Jamie have good disposition magic dust she sprinkles on her Chinese cresteds? Fae is easy and why? Maybe I'll never be sure where the gentle toughness of a good disposition comes from. I never did follow up on meeting Peggy's dad. And I continue to enjoy Pam's without too much thinking about it. It just is. And Fae's just is. And thankful for Jackie to have her. And Jackie is doing well, being Jackie, the good dispositioned street fighter that she is.

That street-fighter peppy disposition served Jackie well in the three jobs she previously held in North Carolina. The first was at the Stop 'n Shop where she fell in love with making hearty deli sandwiches. Once on a visit, I asked her to step out from the cash register to get a "we're heading home now" picture, but Jackie would not step out. The owner had taught these young beach bucks to stay on point at work and she did. "Mom, my friends make as much in one night at the restaurant as I make all week here!" Not being able to keep up with a rough night waiter job, Jackie returned the next summer on the beverage cart during the day at the golf course and got that little pay check right up with her roomies.

Settling down in bill-paying reality, her first real job was in Raleigh. I stopped by her work and the most fun young-for-a-grandma came over to Jackie's work space. I wouldn't forget the lady who wore different outfit-matching wigs every day. She looked at me, the mom, and said, oh yea, Jackie may have been small, may have been young, may have been new in the work world but no mistaking, this girl was a force. She shook her head "no" and then "yes" and I knew what she meant. When Jackie worked, she took ownership, was a force and a mighty one.

After transplant and time went on, that disposition had opportunities to come through. She was the featured guest one week on a podcast called PT Pintcast, tailored for physical therapists, often with guests, patients like Jackie telling them what it was like on her end of the relationship. Be engaged, be empathetic, what Jackie had experienced receiving "PT" and it showed by that successful mobilization we were all witnessing. Just as Jackie sounded on the podcast, she looked on the local morning news segment, "Jackie Price: A Long Road with Cystic Fibrosis."

The newscaster ended saying she didn't even cry. Jackie smiled. Her dad taught her how to look at the good in life, to work out the bad with the help of loved ones, and she did. Jackie was real and when the next newscast happened later in summer, tearful Jackie met her donor's mother.

No Fooling

Maybe people are more like paper. Maybe people are paper. Some of us are three-hole punched, margined, ruled notebook paper, reliable and available. Some sturdy like cardboard, even corrugated, a bit too tough for a people to be. Sandpaper, rough, not so good but they're out there. We all know them and avoid them when we can, though sandpaper does smooth down eventually given the opportunity. Wax paper, computer paper, card stock, all types out there, and assortments.

Jackie reminds me of tissue paper or should I say, Jackie is tissue paper, colorful tissue paper. Mixed with other elements, strong and lively, making for happiness, yet fragile and requiring care. Never know what turn that colorful tissue paper will take, though it will not sit in a three-ring binder and not likely in a file folder. Right now, I'm thinking a file folder would be a quiet place to rest, uneventfully, but instead, I'm mom sitting next to fragile Jackie in hospital recovery after a surgery to clean out synovial fluid in her hip joint that attracted infection and caused pain.

Quirky but on the transplant page, not so quirky. Things looked uncomplicated in there but where this came from, not so uncomplicated. They've figured everything else out so far for this dear work of art. We wait with frayed edges. Jackie's asleep for the moment, will continue to put the collage of her life together. Be the paper that you are with all the scribble, worn edges, folds, tears, and wrinkles that create the work of art that is your life.

Sail Away

Jackie is ready to sail away from the hospital. Her weight is up, she feels better, and the IV medications are working. The doctors want a more specific magic elixir for what more specifically is getting after her hip joint and the doubly difficult lab results aren't back yet. Keeping the blood balanced is apparently a big part of transplant and the chemist in them all is still at work figuring out the correct concoction, err… medication, so in the hospital Jackie remains, but not for long.

That hip joint incision is healing nicely, though orthopedic surgeons may need an afternoon session or two with the plastic surgeons. Dracula bites. So Jackie's there and lucky for her today, a dose of art happiness with "Aunt Bean Artworks." Christine came and taught Jackie some new art techniques. At the hand of this wonderful artist, Jackie is making the art her own and can't wait to sail away home to that collection of art supplies she's building.

Jackie wheel-chaired upon discharge to an evening event in the Physicians' Conference Room in the hospital, an Advanced Lung Disease/Cystic Fibrosis Program meeting of doctors and support staff, patients and families all held together by this crazy world of disease. Jackie spoke. An event long since well-planned, the discharge timing was right. Do what you have to do to the best of your ability and without hesitation was her message that night. Someone in the audience openly cried.

Jackie cooperated with her doctors, she cooperated with her disease. It tried to take her. In life, be ready. Diseases create new definitions and this was a new definition of "ready" and a definition she would share when she could, like that night. She would do the same with her transplant demands, honor and respect and work with them, settling them into their rightful place, and she would share.

No matter what, Jackie would be happy. What causes a person to wake up happy no matter what happens, to enjoy life exponentially no matter what a day might bring, to get behind yet look ahead? A picture of Jackie at a young age remained on our refrigerator. Jackie's lips, always chapped, and the chap would gravitate away from her lips creating its own circle around but away from her mouth. The t-shirt she was wearing in that photograph read, "Attitude is everything." Chapped lips were nothing. Jackie embraced what was before her whether she put it there, someone else put it there, or it put itself there.

Looking back, she embraced her care. I remember when Jackie was ten or eleven, Dr. Clayton said to me, "She's becoming you." And then she entered her teens. She loved her doctors like parents and they ached when she pushed back on her care. I was thankful at age seventeen, her senior year of high school, when Jackie began driving herself to Dr. Williams. Dr. Matthew Williams' adult pulmonologsit visits overlapped with the pediatric visits I still attended. Not my idea, wish I could take credit, but it worked, allowing Jackie to forge, on her own and bravely, her own doctor-patient relationship.

I met Dr. Williams two years after Jackie met him, one year after she left for college. She came home that summer and I took one look at her and knew she needed to be hospitalized. As her mother, I knew her pulmonary functions by merely looking at her face, and for certain that time.

She had lived her freshman year in the freshman dorm like everyone else there, which meant without doing enough care and there she was, at her appointment with Dr. Williams and for the first time, her mom. "Jackie, I won't be able to help you recover but so many times. You have to take care of yourself. I have to put you in the hospital." I thanked him very much, drove home in my separate car and she followed, packed her belongings, and we left for the hospital admission. During that visit, I was a visitor. I had to walk away. If I owned it, she wouldn't. She needed to own it. Jackie interacted with the doctors herself, after all, doctors of adults don't sign up for parents.

Jackie was so mad one day, she forbid us from entering her hospital room. Any slide backwards brought a sense of fear, wondering if she would come around or continue to slide down and away. Her father and I drove over anyhow and waited in the hospital café for her okay to come up to her room.

"Go home, you're wasting your time! Don't you get it? I don't want you here." Unfulfilled, we got to the van in the parking garage and her father who had a runny nose somehow blew a big snot bubble out of one nostril, which I photographed and texted to Jackie's phone.

He was a great icebreaker. Jackie would not admit it but she loved it. The next day, this "adult" on the adult pulmonary unit allowed us in. The following summer, Jackie came home with higher lung functions than when she left the hospital. She went on to live at the beach for two summers, embracing her care, paying her bills, growing further into adulthood.

Her relationship with Dr. Williams was richly dedicated to her successfully completing college and entering the work force. He offered at any point to contact any professor at her university to explain what she had to do every single day to make it to class, to make it in college. He never had to. Jackie embraced her communications with those professors, embraced studying, embraced her sorority and social life, embraced life as Jackie always would.

Not surprising when Jackie's lungs went down that night in June, when that quiet, wicked (I have to call it that) infection overtook her lungs in that all-night battle, Jackie both feebly and frantically called Dr. Williams. He with Jackie would decide whether to intubate, or not. Of course, Dr. Williams knew Dr. Djorkevik and of course Jackie had to be intubated. We were there and from afar, Dr. Williams was there, too.

Then the switch flipped, Dr. Brown replaced Dr. Williams at the helm of Jackie's life. What drives medical care is the part of the disease that creates the ultimate outcome and with cystic fibrosis, it's preferably a lung transplant. As a child, Jackie engaged with her pediatric pulmonologists every three months, often every week, sometimes daily. They, too, clock hundreds of hours with moms, an irreplaceable relationship by no choice.

Our irreplaceable daughter is here because of pediatric pulmonologists, overlapping with and then followed by adult pulmonologists, overlapping and then followed by transplant pulmonologists, Dr. Brown, at the helm of Jackie's life. She knew Jackie's feet were firmly planted on the ground pre-transplant. She knew Jackie would hit the ground running post-transplant. What grounded Jackie?

Bob

~~~~~~~~~

As a small child, Jackie would act out and I would get tense and upset though I did not yell. We would "borrow" Nick and Elizabeth's neighborhood and go trick-or-treating with them to include their grandparents. I always loved when Jackie's brother wanted to make a point, he referenced how things were done "At Nick's House!" I enjoyed that our children enjoyed their house.

One year, their grandfather and I had an opportunity to talk, walking along with our families trick-or-treating in the dark. He commented, "You don't breathe properly" and offered to teach me how to breathe properly. I wanted to say, "Of course I don't breathe properly and I never will." The following year, he offered again to teach me to breathe properly, to visualize calm, to be calm, and I accepted.

From Bob, I learned to be calm with Jackie, to help her along her way in a good way. When Bob died, I had the honor of speaking at his funeral along with four others, all story-filled from funny to serious, and thankful to have had the chance to say one last thank you to Bob for showing me the calm that Jackie so needed. In a big way, our calm and thought-filled home, that's what grounded Jackie.

Jackie had been poked and prodded, and acting out was

her way of getting back at all those needle jabs from "IV starts." Those IVs would "blow" and they'd have to start another one and then another one and goodness leave the girl alone! Now patients get to have these nifty semi-permanent mediports for intravenous medication access.

Six weeks prior to the first "lungiversary," six months after Jackie's transplant discharge, they placed a mediport. Interventional radiology had seen her multiple times in the previous months and relenting to having something attached to her body again was the right thing to do. It could be "de-accessed" leaving a small mound just under the skin just below the collar bone. Then with a painless puncture, a tiny needle attached to an IV connector could be threaded into the nifty little receptor under the skin in the mound. When "accessed," the mediport needed protection but when "de-accessed," not. Jackie maintained that window of opportunity for worry-free bathing.

Being the complicated sort that she was, having developed tolerances for the anesthesia medication they had arranged for the mediport placement procedure, we waited nearly all day for a different medication and an available anesthesiologist. I was knitting by then and Jackie was watching cooking channels and making grocery lists. She was starting work the following day and anticipating what to bring to work for lunch. Nothing changes.

What would, in fact, change was Jackie becoming a part of something big again, other than her own survival. Rising in the morning, pulling out work clothes, giving the make-up mirror a few glances, and stepping out on time to commute to work was invigorating. Her team at Lidl remained flexible and appreciative of the girl who made it back and wanted to be back, the girl who was reclaiming her identity.

Never would Jackie take work for granted, nor would she easily listen to anyone else do so. Work was fun but fun was fun, too.

She and her new mediport, not hooked up to drugs at the time, made their way down south two hours to a bridal shower. They then made their way north two hours for a wedding. With the blessing of her doctors, she traveled with friends by car, and alone by train, one way or another, reclaiming her life. Some friends she had kept close contact with, others she had not seen since back in college -- Jackie in the normal flow.

Charleston

Jackie's plan to celebrate her transplant one year out by taking this trip with friends via plane to Charleston has been long in the making and tremendous pressure has been on the Inova medical team to assure Mise en Place and indeed, the pieces have fallen into proper place.

Jackie is different now, with her full cheeks due to anti-rejection medications and soft voice due to intubation scarring. She's regained her size and her feet are a little wider, disrupting some of those shoes in her closet. Her scars, each symbolizing someone's success at saving her, are fading. Reminders of where we've been, always looking at where we're going.

Serious hospitalization dulls the taste buds, and now approaching June 21, Jackie's sense of taste is back and the seafood along that southern shore, too, is a celebration. She'll come back to the one-year bronchoscopy and biopsy of lung tissue this upcoming week to check for the health of her new lungs, and for rejection. Jackie's different now. She's had a lung transplant. But she's not different: still bright and high-spirited, having a wonderful time in Charleston with her wonderful friends.

CHAPTER FOURTEEN

SUMMER AGAIN

Jackie made her way by plane to see her brother in Boston. He, like us I am sure, noticed the details, the ting, ting, ting sound of Jackie's rapid stir of sweet ice tea, her clickety-clackety shoes down the hallway, her multi-tasking phone and morning TV show and make-up and hair straightener, conversation, toast and jelly all at once.

So when they forged out, it wasn't post-transplant Jackie, it was Jackie. They walked and biked, kayaked, sailed, duck-boat toured, whale-watched, Fenway Park baseball gamed, and Tasty Burgered in Cambridge at the midnight hour. She came home ready to go again.

We met her brother the following weekend at Beth Ann's in Manhattan and I wore the "Stay Strong" bracelet Beth Ann had given me those months ago, to remind her that we had. All I wanted to do at Beth Ann's was sit and stare out of her Manhattan flat across the river to the Brooklyn cityscape. Maybe I was wearing down. Maybe I was able to relax some. Byron and Jackie and Ashley went on their own at the earliest of hours to a Good Morning, America concert in Central Park, where the group One Republic played "I Lived," a song about cystic fibrosis, Jackie is sure prompted by the sign she held up that said, "I lived despite cystic fibrosis. Recycle yourself. Donate life."

From visiting her granddad in the small town of Culpeper an hour away in Central Virginia, to being in DC for the Fourth of July fireworks, Jackie welcomed herself back to life. This summer would not be missed and Jackie herself was keeping everyone updated.

Jackie: Update

Yesterday something amazing happened... I received a letter from my donor's mother. I had mine ready to send after the 4th of July holiday but after receiving hers, I couldn't wait. This was the hardest page and a half I have ever written and it has taken me a year to come up with the right words because "thank you" is not nearly enough. I can't begin to explain the emotions I felt while reading her letter but was so happy to receive it. I now know the angel who watches over me, who gave me life again, is named Samantha. Everyone cherish your time here on earth and tell those you love, that you love them.

Pounce

~~~~~~~~

We walk into Fairfax Hospital. I'm startled. I'm startled that I'm startled. This summer, out and about in the toasty sun, bicycling in cities, restauranting with friends, wardrobing off-line, driving down the drive-way to fun. That once bare stick at the front porch, the wisteria that grew fast up into the eaves thriving as Jackie has thrived, now replaced by more steady and predictable, beautiful and complex passion flow-er, full, in full bloom like Jackie these days.

It's this summer, not last summer. Last summer in a box in a box, in a hospital in an ICU. Lest I forget, in yet another box, yes in a bed. The bed, confining and liberating. Where some die, where Jackie lived, first by machine and medical mind, by sheer will, time, and miracle if you believe in them.

We're here now... again... not as "Inpatient" but under "Observation Services," an overnight stay af-ter surgically closing the hole in Jackie's stomach, the entry point of nutritional formula, tube feedings. I never liked that... feedings. Over the ten plus years, I called it "night nutrition," slow dripped over several hours directly into the stomach in addition to nor-mal eating during the day, boosting the body's ability to fight off infection due to the cystic fibrosis. Gone now, no need for that boost due to renewed health due to the lung transplant. Why not pop new lungs in these patients preventatively? A pulmonologist once said, a lung transplant is not elective surgery.

Over a year now since this not-elective surgery, mi-nus those months in ICU, the point when the respon-sibility became ours. Every night, no sugarplums dancing in my head, more like medical this, medi-cal that dancing in my head. The dry cough, kidney function, medication management, blood draws, transplant: complex.

It's a lifestyle that calms over time and acts up some. Fortitude is not free. Worry, like filling up those little candy dispensers, lift the head, often Popeye's, eat one of those tart little rectangles, then another. Keep filling the Pez. Like worry, put it away! Sleep. Another tomorrow, a full life, full of anticipation, the good news of a successful lung transplant.

They're still here for Jackie. These are her relationships at this hospital. This is what we worked for and wanted and got. Jackie's weight is back, her strength, near balance, her shoe love fulfilled. We'll leave in the morning after "the bronch," after they put Jackie to sleep… again… and check her lungs… again. There's a little place in the upper airway in question. And always checking for rejection, always in question.

Worry is no way to live so we won't. Odds are in all of our favor as we wander around this world full of lurkings, that which "hides around corners" and tries to take us out. We thrive anyhow, most of us most of the time. Jackie thrives anyhow.

She leaves on a stretcher and I take the visitor's elevator down to Pulmonary Diagnostics, mentally stumbling, physically stumbling, someone in front of me. "Oh, excuse me," I smile. Stop it! That was then. It's now and the sun is toasty and Jackie is twenty-five and living again as twenty-five year olds should, bicycling through cities, restauranting with friends, wardrobing off-line, working, laughing, playing, doing her medical care as they expect. Everyone here smiles. Their success. Jackie's success. I leave the elevator, graciously. Oh sweet success.

Jackie goes home from the hospital and rests well

and then pounce, wakes up with a fever. Undergoing surgery on her stomach was a hit to her system, that gnawing little spot on her upper lung, pneumonia. A reminder that Jackie is still fragile so I'll nurture her through this as mothers do, her medical team will problem-solve her through this as medical teams do.

No more coffee leaking through her gastric tummy hole because it's closed now and she'll recover again from a pneumonia hiccup. Her dog, her car, her sweet bedroom waiting in her certainly-not-perfect-but-loving home, family and friends awaiting her return, that bundle of love. I tell my husband again, "Honey, I feel so lucky."

We did need family and Jackie loved the sauce out of her family. Though too small and too quiet, her family and their crab feasts and potlucks were a bundle of fun for the fun junkie. Jackie's Uncle George had trekked up to the hospital every Monday no matter how hard it was to enter that place. From his home in Luray two hours away, he and Jackie would continue to communicate weekly by phone. Her Aunt Anne had stayed with us that hard summer and stuck with us over the months of pain and progress. She was the one over the years who toted the nail salon up to the hospital for some afternoon diversion every time Jackie was "in."

Josh had swooped into the ICU between cracks of time in his hedge fund job and girlfriend's condo renovation. Christie had come and come again, bringing "normal food" forays and stories of her primary school students. Cousins were threads of normalcy during those fantastical hospital days and will always and evermore be.

Jackie's grandfather learning of her emergency double lung transplant was hard. Having been a criminal lawyer for fifty years, he'd seen so much and our tense and tearful faces calmed when I slipped away to spend time with him once along the way and told him everything would be okay. Granddad did come to the hospital once difficult as it was for him to make his way down the corridor, past the fountain, up the elevator, around and back to the ICU, difficult as it was for him to physically see the predicament we were in and the long way still to go getting out.

Grandma

Have you ever known anyone who reminds you of your mother? After a year-long battle with lung cancer, my mother died. Jackie reminds me of my mother. My mother was effortlessly organized unlike most of us, getting there but never quite. Her finances, time management, eating habits, her physical space, clothing closet and personal belongings, all easily in order. Even her relationships were not messy. Her checkbook was balanced. She did not misplace keys. Meals were meals and snacks were snacks. Early was on time and on time was late. Organized. She just was and Jackie just is.

So when Jackie's doctors say she manages a complex medical regimen with seeming effortlessness, I know why. When I watch Jackie fill up her weekly medication organizer, multiple pill bottles, one pill along this row, two pills every other that way, three or three and a half pills back here again, filling, refilling, continuing, discontinuing, and then add in medical appointments, tests and procedures -- a lot to manage.

I watch Jackie's eyes as she's thinking through all of this and I see my mother sitting there across the table, that pause, that look, the head tilt, hand gestures, the getting it done and getting it right. There's a continued quiet comfort and pleasure in seeing a little of my mother in Jackie.

Jackie spent a lot of childhood time with grandma. They both enjoyed together, apart, together time. They would work on something together like a puzzle, then go off separately and one would read, the other play dolls, then together again back to the puzzle. My mother once found the perfect greeting card: why grandparents and grandchildren were in such harmony, the reason, they have the same common enemy. They both thought that was funny, their own inside joke, we got it but they got it more. My mother and Jackie shared a similar and appreciated sense of humor, so their common enemy enjoyed them both and continues to enjoy seeing the mother now gone in the daughter still here. Being a common enemy is quite nice.

Revealings

Each day can be defined as a revealing. Sometimes at night, hopefully not at night. Wake up one morning, the mayor is arrested. Another morning, he's given a chance at rejoining the community, sitting on his own couch, eating from his own refrigerator. One day, visit a small town courthouse and find a Confederate marker all edgy about "the War of Northern Aggression" and wonder when that will be taken down. Another day, come to find out, maybe all of the Confederate markers will be taken down.

Each day, a revealing of what was left unknown the day before. We got a recent revealing. It's Jackie's hip. As if it wasn't enough to wake up one day a few weeks ago to find out "tissue paper" Jackie needed that hip joint washed out to clear out infection. Didn't plan to know about that sort of procedure. And now revealed by the most recent MRI, Magnetic Resonance Imaging, that the ball of the hip joint has become necrotic, meaning a blood supply loss in the process of being sick with infection and taking transplant medications. This is called a revealing for an old person, not for a young person.

Along with the hip revealing, there's another. Jackie is now listed for a kidney transplant as her kidney function fell into the kidney transplant range, managed now by medications and not dialysis. Once the kidney function falls below 20%, patients are listed for a transplant and remain listed, even if the function percent climbs up again.

Kidneys are rulers of the roost, in case you didn't know what your own kidneys are. Jackie's kidney function is somewhat back up so we can ignore the kidney transplant list revealing and stick with finding out what orthopedics has to say about her hip. It's a mood killer. But those revealings that put us in a bad mood are not like the "You're not going to live on the planet earth anymore" kind that people get, not us.

Plenty of happy revealings are out there and I'd like to think the ones that aren't happy lose their standing in time. Jackie keeps being hooked up to things like IV antibiotics for a touch of pneumonia since she's immunosuppressed, and to a blood sugar monitor since transplant drugs fuss with blood sugar levels. She's not yet a year out of the hospital and the revealing one day that she's getting her life back not attached to something medical remains in view, so many of the harder revealings behind her. May that sense of impatience pass. May we be willing and grateful, and ever-loving.

We met the kidney transplant surgeon after the kidney function percent drop signaled us to do so. He was new there, and informative. Though it was best to meet him, it was also best not to need him. He thought Jackie's two kidneys had quit on her and he was ready to put one new one in. Not yet.

Lung transplant surgeries are much more complicated but the donor match is much less complicated. There aren't living lung donors since taking one lung from a live donor is too compromising. Kidney transplant surgeries are much less complicated but the donor match is much more complicated. Those who need a kidney only need one and those donating a kidney only need one. Kidney donors can be live or deceased. More kidneys are available due to the sad state of opioid use taking so many of our young people. Those drugs hurt livers but not kidneys.

Being listed means willing donors can be screened and moms are often a good match. Jackie would benefit mentally from having that kidney waiting in her back pocket, so I began the climb towards the comprehensive medical clearance to become her donor. Did I need to worry about the psych. evaluation? Probably not but "cracking" in the middle of that interview piece did cross my mind. These sorts of situations can turn people into what they don't want to be and maybe I would break down or act out, opposites but similar and neither desirable.

I learned that donating a kidney can result in temporary feelings of loss. I imagine the voluntarily removal of a part of the body, no body-benefit to the donor, would result in some deep psychic feeling of loss and maybe finally reading the book, *Necessary Losses* would help though I never read the book, *Parenting Is Not For Cowards* because I always said as a reading teacher by trade, sometimes reading the title is enough. I didn't want to be a cowardly parent. I don't want to mishandle necessary losses.

The transplant social worker pointed out, best to know these things to avoid surprises. No surprises. Right down my alley. Any warning of any unexpected challenges would be a whole lot better than the challenges we'd faced without warning. This all has led me to believe that Jackie gaining a kidney if need be, gaining a new body part that works well, would be a gain for her mentally, as well, and we all know that would make me happy.

Even with all this togetherness, Jackie and I were getting along well. Home care had long since become routine and manageable as long as we remembered Jackie was an adult. The balance between reminding her of something important she may have overlooked and telling her what to do or planning how she should do it remained on my mind. Letting go of the mom who raised Jackie and embracing the mom who could leave being in charge of Jackie up to Jackie wasn't always perfectly executed.

I loved sinus washes over the years. That mix of warm

water and salt was such a clean and simple way to clear nasal congestion. Jackie hated them. I suppose what was most unhelpful was the pediatric ear, nose, and throat specialist recommending this nasal attachment to the dental device called a "water flosser." The motorized pump caused a stream of pressurized, pulsating water to flow from this reservoir through, not a dental tip but rather a nasal tip reaching difficult recesses in the nose. It worked like drowning a swamp rat. I rapidly let go of that idea.

Of all the care she endured due to her cystic fibrosis, she knew sinus washes were the negotiable ones so when she got mad, she would say, "I'm not doing my sinus washes!" That one, she could win. Even to this point, I don't bring up sinus washes much and look the other way with hopes that she does them and loves doing them like I want her to.

Jackie's life has always been intermingled with up-ups and downs. I think about the song, "The Dance," famously sung by Garth Brooks. "Looking back… on the memory of… the dance we shared… beneath the stars above. For a moment all the world was right" except I wish the song-writer would change the part about saying "goodbye." I understand, "Now I'm glad I didn't know the way it all would go." It is true that "our lives are better left to chance. I could have missed the pain but I'd have to miss the dance," as well as, "Holding you, I held everything" but "everything" can and should be about moving on together.

The truth is, Fae is the one I hold and hug the most. Wanting to hug Jackie too much, Fae is squishy and huggable like Jackie so Fae gets most of the holding and hugging. Jackie prefers virtual hugs and she gets lots of those and just the right amount of embrace hugs from the mom of a near-twenty-six year old.

Hans, a friend of Jackie's from college and an artist, painted a beautiful watercolor of lungs made of pink roses with roses all around, sixty-five of them for "sixty-five roses," the name for cystic fibrosis given long ago by a little boy who had it and didn't understand what his disease was called. T-shirts adorned with that beautiful painting helped raise money to offset the medical cost of life now associated with not the disease but the transplant.

The Kitchen Table

So much more goes on here other than eating. Sitting here now with no place to go. It's been a long time and I won't take it for granted. I glance over: laying across the back of Jackie's cushioned chair at the end is a black t-shirt with white letters across the front, LXV, those "sixty-five roses," cystic fibrosis, ever a part of our lives.

I've heard Jackie sitting here communicating with other people she's connecting with, miles away, but close by age and interests, by this disease, and by lung transplant. They have a lot in common like embracing what has happened and making plans to move forward. They sound tough and sure and able. Over-comers do find each other and I feel fortunate to share this kitchen table with one of them. Jackie's "Donate Life" license plate reads as if so simple, "NU-LUNGS."

When I glance back to my up-lifted laptop computer at my place, a small window pops up in the top right corner, "CareFirst: Your EOB." Explanation of Benefit. I haven't kept up but the truth is, BlueCross/

BlueShield has kept up. I once reminded the lady at the hospital door, the one with the BlueCross transition home folder, "We're your ambassadors, cheaper than advertising." My witness to their role in Jackie's success will not go unnoticed. Still, chunks leave my paycheck each month for the privilege of belonging. I was a teacher for more than one reason. I glance at my computer for more than one reason. Jackie is on the news.

The Bracelet

"Family Meets Recipient of Late Daughter's Lungs NBC4"

Google brings up a news segment dated September 11, 2017, Jackie and her donor's mother meeting last weekend. On Jackie's wrist is a bracelet, an Ankh in gold, the Egyptian hieroglyph for "Breath of Life." John of Personal Touch Jewelers, a gem in our community for thirty years, is an artist who is also a jeweler.

I brought to him gold from various pieces belonging to my mother who had passed away, looking for a meaningful connection to her by jewelry. John was wearing this Ankh bracelet he had made for himself a long time back. "I want that," I told him. John created his bracelet twice again, for me and for Jackie. Jackie wears hers everywhere she goes.

Every so often, my phone rings and it's John. He's thinking about Jackie and wants to know. I think about the bracelets and try not to cry, try not to tell him too much because it's too much, though I don't think he thinks so. It's just that the bracelet, that gold, and the story that I brought into his store that day, the artist in him. The bracelet is more than the sum of each part, more than a bracelet, and a sweet side story showing up on the news recording that "Personal Touch" night.

Our family met Jackie's donor family that evening in September when Jackie's brother could be in town, fifteen months after we learned of Samantha's passing. The letters exchanged between Samantha's mother and Jackie were grippingly similar. Meeting them was grippingly charming. We left the television cameras and the Greater Washington Transplant Community office and had dinner together. Angela cried the whole night and hugged Jackie the whole night. She said hearing and feeling a part of her daughter helped her move on. They say most families don't meet, one or the other never responds to the letter but our families responded and met and will stay in contact.

All Five Senses

Love is about all five senses. Maybe some of ours are half asleep. Maybe our awareness is what's half asleep. The sense of smell, the strongest, I think walking into Jackie's bedroom, the scent of Jackie when Jackie's not there. Who notices? Moms of babies notice, moms of children who have died notice, and lovers newly in love. We don't notice but we should. The sense of smell becomes familiar and we forget but I think, in fact, our sense of smell does remember, something we should not forget.

When Jackie was intubated and at once silenced, such a longing arose, such a love through the sense of hearing. I listen now to Jackie's voice, pause at all the sounds to notice and to remember, going back in time, the familiar early on and through the years held dear. Those sounds, when taken away and given back, love resonated.

Touch irreplaceably connects us to each other. Jackie doesn't want mountainous hugs from her mother by now but throughout her hospital stay, her mother's touch was daily and healing and important to us both. When Jackie was little, she used to say, "Mom, you're squishing me!" So her nickname was "Squishy." I imagine a lot of people have the nickname "Squishy." Thankful we are.

I glanced over at Jackie once long ago driving across town to a soccer game. "Stop looking at me, mom! You even love my feet!" I did from the very beginning love those little cornrow nuggets for toes. Once, as well, I placed this two inch green ceramic frog at the base of the river birch at the top of our driveway to see how long before Jackie's dad noticed it. He drove up that evening and came into the house and asked me first who put that ceramic frog there. I've learned a lot from my husband's sense of observation, looking and seeing, and love even more because of it.

How do we love by taste? The sense of taste and love, I've come to believe, are bridged together by food. Maybe a food fest is also a love fest. Our family always through the years enjoyed nightly dinnertime and when Byron flies home, our dinners together are most important. When he's gone, Jackie phones her brother on speaker to "join us for dinner." Truly one of Jackie's greatest joys in her recovery is meals with people she loves. Food is love by taste.

May we wake up and love with all five senses.

Jackie's 26th birthday ould soon arrive. "9/16/91." In the medical world, those numbers provide stiff competition for a person's name as the identifier. How many times had I stated those numbers in the past months? Nine sixteen ninety-one. Hundreds of times and I plan to repeat it hundreds of times more, and Jackie will too. Jackie spent her birthday with friends as young adults do. She expected little, believing we had given her so much, art lessons at The Art League in Old Town Alexandria, a happy place for a happy girl though her hip was bothering her at the potter's wheel.

The art teacher knew enough about Jackie to accommodate missed lessons due to medical interruptions Jackie had to deal with. We had been told that number of days in the ICU times five happens to be the recovery index. Four months times five meant twenty months and that would bring us to Jackie's recovery, to her second lungversary, still nine months away and that would be okay. The enormity of the ICU experience looming in the background brought us down for a smooth landing with any challenges we would meet.

Cookout

Jackie is not feeling well. I'm not sure if she is sick but

we will find out today. Waiting in the transplant out-patient exam room for her trusted Dr. Brown. Jackie's not hungry, she's tired, and the pneumonia in her upper lung area has not completely cleared. Recovery is winding and hilly though by definition, less winding and less hilly over time.

Jackie got on with her life and spent the long week-end away from home relaxing with friends, returning to an empty house as her parents went to a Labor Day cook out, a pachamonchu, which is a Bolivian cooking event involving red hot rocks, banana leaf-wrapped raw meat, and potatoes buried in the ground for a few hours. Glad they knew what they were doing.

Being on texting checking on Jackie, this was the place to be. The Bolivian people are deeply joyous, unhurried, what I needed to be yesterday. I got lost yesterday, still thinking about my sweet girl, listening, not understanding but enjoying the inside-out outside-in beauty of the Spanish language. They spoke to us in English, even still.

Even still, I was able to be there and not be there, which is the way it is these days. I keep my phone close at hand, my link to Jackie. There's no good time to talk or call people back these days. There's no good time to go to a cookout but we went and glad we did. And now Jackie and I are in the doctor's office and glad we are.

Yesterday of the thirty or so hovering over that dirt pit filled with cooking meat and potatoes and then hours later eating amazing food, we sat down next to someone with two grown children. She said, as I noticed that thin vertical scar at the base of her neck, "A trach." She's had a tracheotomy. She's been through something. Then she tells me.

A black ice car accident close to home put her in a coma in an ICU. I briefly mentioned Jackie. She briefly mentioned her daughter, majoring now in Art after losing a year of college fighting cancer. Months lost, a life gained. I looked across the way to her husband. He was laughing, and smiling. He's been through something. I knew. He got to keep his family of four, too. She and I talked further as kindred souls do, ate delicious food, and we left for home. Time for us to nurture Jackie and find out today what next. Better go. The doc just walked in.

Maybe it was the recovery process sputtering along and the need for rest. Jackie presented better than expected. Dr. Brown adjusted her medications and we rode home and further down the road to recovery. Then we hit a bump and kind of a big one. It was Jackie's nagging hip.

Jackie: Hip Reflections

After the initial shock of finding out I had a double lung transplant, I was excited. I made plans to run for miles and go on long hikes in the mountains. These are things I had so badly wanted to be able to do but couldn't due to coughing spells and feeling out of breath due to cystic fibrosis. With new lungs and the ability to breathe again, I have gratefully made plans and accomplished some of them. But due to an array of complications, I physically can't accomplish running miles or hiking mountains right now.

Namely, the medications that saved my life have harmed my hip joint. It acts up badly these days and eventually will need to be replaced. Yes, a hip replacement and I'm only 26 years old, but I am going to look at that as small stuff after all of the big stuff I've been through. As human beings we have a tendency to initially focus on the negatives, what we don't have but want or think we need but can't get. We all have to bring our minds around to think that in time, things fall into place, think about all that we CAN do and all of the ways life has compensated us.

Stories often circle back and this medical one did. Dr. Katugaha fought successfully to eradicate the fungal infection that gripped Jackie's old lungs. It found its way into that deteriorated hip joint. So rare, with little or perhaps no point of reference, Dr. K forged on to eradicate this remnent of the past found in that hip which in the future will be replaced.

CHAPTER FIFTEEN

AND INTO AUTUMN

Crisp, clear autumn brought crisper, clearer breathing, and thinking. Jackie started a blog sharing her way of looking at the world, sharing her optimism, explaining her disease process, more current and recurrent medical challenges, and some of the dreams she had while under, the vividness, almost too twisted and gnarled to explain. Jackie is finding a way.

She's posted her wild "Mountain Mama, take me home Country Roads" video produced from a mountain weekend in West Virginia. She's posted Blue's Mount Everest endeavor to raise money for herself and for her friend's father with cancer. Steven Blue is a friend of Jackie's from college and since then, she and her dad send him recorded messages, her dad singing, "My Boy Blueooooo!" I can't keep up.

Pink and grey spot-bellied Fae, the dog with long beautiful hair, a mane down her back and bell-bottomed dog hair feet, hippy that she is, runs slippedly-slide, lickety-split, scrambling when Jackie walks in the door. That seven-and-a-half pound little pony girl stays close, even by the toilet as the obsessed sometimes do. She lounges on the bed as Jackie sorts through her masterful wardrobe and comes down with Jackie for long, slow dinners with mom and dad followed by remote chats with her brother. Fae follows over to the art table where Jackie gets lost in Zentangles. They'll rest together and then Happy Jackie is out again.

Balance

Our aim has always been about balance, not to tip the balance. After college, Jackie and her brother and Christine spent a month roaming through Europe. I received texts. Jackie wanted to taxi, Byron wanted to walk. Jackie wanted fabulous food, Byron economical food. She wanted to get to bed, he to stay out late, twenty minutes in museums for her, half a day for him. I asked them what Jesus would do.

I've always said "balance" is my favorite word and I've always said "balance" is Jesus' favorite word, too. They got it and went on in some semblance of balance, letting go of the bickering. For us, always seeking balance, in connection to body and mind, and relationships.

Keith Whitley, a musician who died in 1989, sang a well-known song called "When You Say Nothing at All." The lyrics are some of my favorites though not the title. My premise would be that saying just enough, reaching that balance between saying too much and saying nothing at all, is the sweet spot. Nonetheless, the lyrics held in marrying Jackie's dad in the eighties. "It's amazing how you can speak right to my heart…The smile on your face lets me know that you need me, the truth in your eyes saying you'll never leave me, a touch of your hand says you'll catch me if ever I fall."

I wonder if Don Schlitz and Paul Overstreet struggled to create these words as I have struggled with some of my written words, or if they came easily as some of mine have. My favorite line is, "Old Mister Webster could never define, what's being said between your heart and mine" and I suppose if hearts speak, this song's lyrics speak to the balance of love between all of us in this family.

Not Then, Now

I open our front door, "The Breathing Shop" label rests on top of the box. We need a breathing shop? Masks Jackie may need, nebulizer treatments to combat a little cough. The cough persists. The cough, not so little. We find out, not her lungs. Jackie won't need the nebulizer.

A snatch of one of those buggies up in that nose, that sweet little devilish nose, buggies her dad wants for catfish bait, sent rather to the Inova laboratory. Another box, "Thermosafe Insulated Shipper: temperature sensitive product, every degree matters," home IV antibiotics to combat infection.

Jackie needs sinus surgery, again. Her temperature rises, again. She's admitted, again. Her ENT, ear nose and throat doctor, again. We're feeling good about sinus surgery this time, a power wash in the schnook that gave her trouble before, giving her trouble again.

Down to the donut-planked table, hospital CAT scan area again. I wait in the hallway next to the big case of daggers, marked "air clean systems, the fume control experts." Thankful we don't need daggers and thankful clean air matters in this "Patient Holding" area, more like mother holding area. I'm not going to get upset in spite of the "external disaster plan now in effect" drill announcement we hear coming down the corridor. There will be no internal or external disasters this time. Diseases have a mind of their own and Jackie's sinuses still have cystic fibrosis, not a disaster.

Three hours in, Dr. Ravi Swamy who operated on Jackie's nose the last time, willing to operate on it again, comes out. I wait and try not to remember in spite of the fact that my mind works in reruns. Good news: the surgery, more extensive than expected, went well. Good news, Jackie's new lungs, healthy, can take it.

Good news, we can handle the sinus surgery aftermath. Jackie calls across to my chair-bed, four a.m. "Mom, it's happening again. Just like last time. This is how it started last time, all this bleeding. It's happening again."

I could have been there all night long helping Jackie every minute with bleeding and congestion and discomfort, but that one chance to pull out of that unfriendly bed chair and go to her, the reason to be there. "No, Jackie, it's not like last time. Last time we were being transferred to the ICU at four a.m. This is now and this is how it's supposed to go."

I'm wearing my earrings this time because I know

234 of JAN PRICE

Jackie will soon be wearing her earrings to that Chili Cook-Off next weekend, and the bracelet, the ankh, the symbol of breathing, of life. My mind remembers where the car is in this complex complex. I'm knitting, Jackie's reading. Jackie's sending me down to the Park Ave Café for Ruebens and the occasional server who does not know me still asks if I work here. The bandana rag on my head, jean jacket, and shirttail hanging out, not a clue as my face is so familiar. Jackie's medical team, far from strangers now, still working hard because diseases are hard and Jackie is still complicated. But she's done well and she is well. And our girl will be home again soon.

This year that's now followed Jackie's bilateral lung transplant hospital discharge has been full of good news and other news. Compared to what? Keeping the old lungs? Having no lungs? Having new lungs that required our care? Thus far, no acute rejection, increased lung functions, and deep and cleansing breaths.

They still can't believe, the girl who was living her life back then, living it completely in spite of those bad lungs that wouldn't make it. They still can't believe, the girl now meeting this complex medical demand with new lungs and enjoying her life. Those good lungs, truly the champion of this story, tied for first with Jackie and her good medical team, good stewards of those good lungs. "Champion." Her brother was right.

Jackie has things to say and to do, participating with the Cystic Fibrosis Foundation and Washington Regional Transplant Community. She continues endless socializing, and art and writing, too. I continue writing by way of paper scraps. It's done something good, helped me to cope, allowed me to think, to rely on others, and brought forth the positive, and it will for Jackie. Maybe that's what writing does and just so happens, the reader benefits. The writer, the reader, we all benefit.

Jackie looks well and she is well. She manages diabetes, washed in with the transplant drugs and maybe will wash out along with some of the other side effects we hope to rid. Jackie is listed for the kidney transplant possibly sometime out in time and possibly not at all, should those sturdy deals continue to cooperate. She needs that hip replaced, more hospital, more specialists, more special people. Jackie's special. Her father says we're all special and thankful we're here fitting in that category of alive and well, and special.

I look at Jackie. Is she here because of me, her father, because of Dr. Brown, Dr. King, Dr. Clayton, all the people who answered the phone when we made medical appointments over the years, the ones who called back with test results or mailed medical records from one specialist to another? Is she here because of the gastroenterologist, the otolaryngologist, the radiologist, the endocrinologist? Is she here because of Jackie, smart and determined, and that strong will to live?

What did save Jackie's life those months ago in Inova Fairfax Hospital's Heart and Vascular Institute were surely the far reaches of medical science. People like Jackie stretch those limits, bringing the next set of limits in medical science in reach. We've suffered, we've given, and we've gained. This happened to a family, it happened to a mom, it happened to a young girl and shouldn't have, but it did.

I always say, "This is the only life you will ever get, the only body you will ever have. You are a whole person no matter what. You deserve the utmost care and respect. We will see you through." My friend, Val, said reading my writing made her cry, reading Jackie's writing makes her smile. Jackie now has a voice and to the world, she has a lot to say. I'll put this writing away, read it again later, and send it out into the world. Jackie is now out in the world. The life of a daughter, our daughter, goes on. God bless those titanium ovaries.

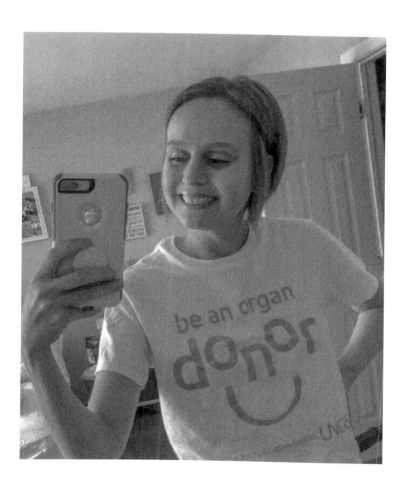

To contact Jackie and view color images of her journey:

Blog: www.pricelessbreaths.com
Instagram: pricelessbreaths
Facebook public group: Priceless Breaths
Email: pricelessbreaths@gmail.com

Jackie's Transplant Medical Team
Inova Fairfax Hospital Heart and Vascular Institute

Dr. A. Whitney Brown, MD
Director Clinical Operations Advanced Lung Disease and Transplant Program Director of the Adult Cystic Fibrosis and Bronchiectasis Program

Adam Cochrane, PharmD, MPH
Transplant Pharmacist

Dr. Andrew D. Howard, MD, FACP
Metropolitan Nephrology Associates

Dr. Shalika Katugaha, MD, FACP
Medical Director Transplant Infectious Disease

Dr. Christopher King, MD, FACP, FCCP
Medical Director Transplant and Advanced Lung Disease Critical Care Program

Lauren Marinak, MSN, NP-C
Transplant Nurse Practitioner

Medical Doctors also in Jackie's Story

Dr. James E. Clayton, MD
Pediatric Lung and Allergy Center

Dr. Heidi Dalton, MD, MCCM
Medical Director Adult and Pediatric Extracorporeal Life Support Program

Dr. Svetolik Djurkovic, MD
Medical Director Medical Critical Care Services

Dr. Sandeep Khandhar, MD
Medical Director Thoracic Surgery

Dr. Amit "Bobby" Mahajan, MD, FCCP, DAABIP
Medical Director Interventional Pulmonology

Dr. Charles Murphy, MD, CPPS
Medical Director Cardiovascular Intensive Care Unit

Dr. John Osborn, MD, FAAP
Director of Pediatric Pulmonary Medicine
Swedish Medical Center, Seattle, Washington

Adam M. Pearlman, MD
Metropolitan Nephrology Associates

Dr. Liam Ryan, MD
Thoracic and Cardiac Surgery, Transplant Surgery

Dr. Ravi S. Swamy, MD, MPH, ENT
Metropolitan ENT

Dr. Erik Teicher, MD, FACS
Surgical Critical Care, Trauma Surgery

Dr. Matthew D. Williams, MD
Northern Virginia Pulmonology and Critical Care Associates, P.C.

We thank all of the many doctors and nurses over the years who
have brought wellness to our family.

77627440R00135

Made in the USA
Middletown, DE
23 June 2018